Torn

A Simple Guide to ACL Tears and Healing for Girls

Joy Werner and Doug Werner

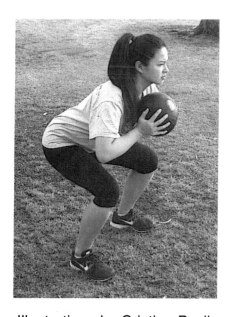

Illustrations by Cristina Byvik

Special contribution by Dr. Justin Balleza

Edited by Phyllis Carter

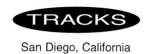

San Diego, California

Torn

A Simple Guide to ACL Tears and Healing for Girls
Joy Werner and Doug Werner

Tracks Publishing
140 Brightwood Avenue
Chula Vista, CA 91910
619-476-7125
tracks@cox.net
www.startupsports.com
trackspublishing.com

Publisher's Cataloging-in-Publication

Werner, Joy (Joy X.), 1997-

   Torn : a simple guide to ACL tears and healing for girls / Joy Werner and Doug Werner ; illustrations by Cristina Byvik ; special contribution by Dr. Justin Balleza ; edited by Phyllis Carter. -- San Diego, California : Tracks, [2015]

      pages : illustrations ; cm.

      ISBN: 978-1-935937-69-2
      Includes bibliographical references and index.
      Summary: Torn is the story of author Joy Werner's struggle with two anterior cruciate ligament (ACL) injuries over the course of 24 months. ACL tears are serious knee injuries that plague youth sport, particularly young female athletes, and this book describes the long journeys of healing that the injuries demand, including the emotional and mental challenges. The personal perspective is supported by general information about the ACL, ACL injuries, and treatment. Torn is not only a guide but a real-world tale of what a young athlete had to endure and overcome when confronted with ACL injuries. It will be helpful to the thousands of young people and their families who face this trauma each year.--Publisher.

      1. Anterior cruciate ligament--Wounds and injuries. 2. Anterior cruciate ligament--Wounds and injuries--Treatment. 3. Anterior cruciate ligament--Surgery. 4. Knee--Wounds and injuries. 5. Knee--Wounds and injuries--Treatment. 6. Knee--Surgery. 7. Sports injuries. 8. Sports injuries --Treatment. 9. Sports injuries in children. 10. Sports injuries in children-- Treatment. 11. Women athletes--Wounds and injuries. I. Werner, Doug, 1950- II. Byvik, Cristina. III. Balleza, Justin. IV. Carter, Phyllis (Phyllis Ortiz), 1942- V. Title.

RD561 .W47 2015   2015908543
617.5/82044--dc23   1508

For My Mother,
Kathleen Wheeler

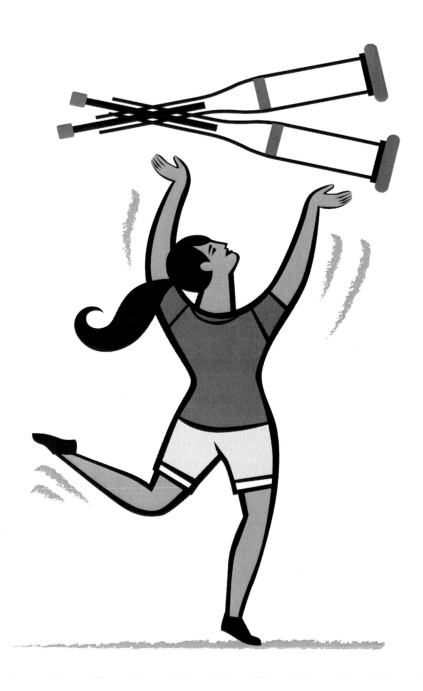

Contents

We never know how high we are
Till we are called to rise;
And then, if we are true to plan,
Our statures touch the skies.

Emily Dickinson

Badge
One girl's story

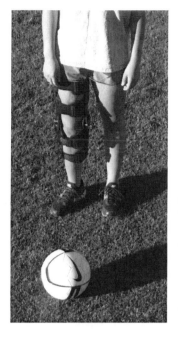

Torn is the story of one girl's experience with and recovery from two ACL tears over the course of about two years.

That's right, *two* ACL injuries — *on the same knee.* Her right knee is beaded with surgical imprints we have come to acknowledge as battle scars — her badge of courage.

The book includes personal viewpoints from Joy and her father as well as a variety of (easily digested) technical information. The latter includes particulars about ACL injury, reconstruction and rehabilitation, especially as it relates to young female athletes.

The personal reflections are probably the most important parts of the book because they are personal. When you get hurt this badly you want to hear authentic voices. Someone like yourself who can tell you all about it. Others suffering from knee injury will relate to the personal accounts and learn from the technical information that has been edited for easy reading.

When we say technical we mean facts and figures and explanations. The sort of thing you can fish up for yourself on the internet. But we've filtered it out OUR WAY, and the results are understandable and (hopefully) a bit more interesting than the typical ACL article.

Here's the idea (and our claim to worthiness): the reader will discover another resource outside the doctor's office and the welter of online information that may seem distant, formal and somewhat incomprehensible.

Doc will fix you, but he or she is still a medical professional and as such conveys a certain detachment born of inside knowledge, talent and experience. Some of these people are race-horses — thoroughbreds who live for the surgical event and the miracle of reconstruction. And that's a good thing. You want your surgeon to be talented and ever so confident — no doubt about that. But what they see every day is something you endure just once (with any luck) and besides, it's your knee.

And how could we forget? The book is loaded with exercises. Exercises to rehab the knee. Exercises to strengthen the core. Exercises to strengthen the legs. Exercises to enhance athletic movement.

If nothing else, here's an illustrated guide of training tasks for knee rehabilitation and general athletic prowess for young female athletes. The latter are most important because they are designed to prevent injury to the knee in the first place!

OK, dig in. And remember, if you've suffered a torn ACL, it does get better.

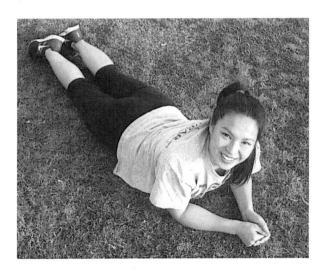

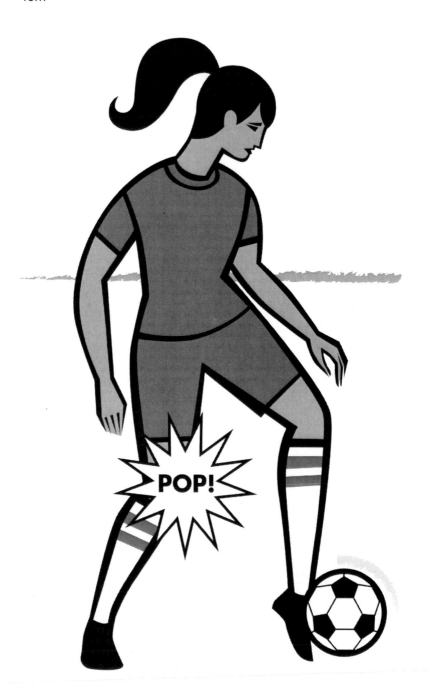

1. *It is what it is*

Joy's notes

Crunch

It was the first few minutes of the first game of State Cup. After a bit I received the ball and immediately a defender was on me. I made a move to break free, but I heard a POP and felt a CRUNCH in my knee. Next thing I knew I was holding my knee in a fetal position in a world of pain. A warm feeling surged into my hurt leg. I knew something was wrong, of course, but I didn't know how wrong.

> I knew something was wrong, of course, but I didn't know how wrong.

I was escorted off the field and asked if I needed medical attention and with little hesitation said YES. The first aider provided by the event looked me over and said that she didn't think it was major, meaning my ACL. Perhaps, she said (along with others, including coach) it was a torn meniscus that would heal on its own in time. I was thinking I just had a tumble and I'd be fine if I just shook it off. After 10 minutes on the bench, I felt better and the pain began to go away. I jumped up and started doing sprints to warm up so that I could get back into the game. After all, it was semi-finals!

But as soon as I ran back onto the field and started playing again, I KNEW that there was a serious problem. My knee was buckling as if it wasn't even connected. I could barely crawl off the field. After the buckling, I didn't want to hear what the medic had to say. I wanted to see a bona fide doc and find out EXACTLY what the problem was.

Even though there was no reason to think so, I felt as though I had let my dad down. I felt embarrassed. Like I failed. I don't know why I felt this way and even now I can't explain why.

At this point I thought my injury would take some time to heal, but that I'd be back pretty soon. That night our team stayed in a hotel where we tore through the halls, horsed around in the rooms and went up and down the elevators. Even though my knee hurt and I was (sort of) icing it, I still tried to keep up — I didn't want to miss out on the fun! Soon my knee swelled up and turned a kind of blackish blue color. In the middle of the night I got up to go to the bathroom and when I touched the floor I almost fell because I was in so much pain and unable to support my own weight.

Next morning I was really wobbling around. Because our team had lost the last game we headed home to San Diego. Throughout the ride I was worried about the extent of my injury, but I remained hopeful that it would heal in a few weeks. I had NO IDEA what was to come. When we finally got home, my mom was super worried about me. I just wanted to go see a doctor and get an MRI. I think one of the worst parts of any mishap like this is the anticipation of finding out what's wrong.

But it DID NOT get better. The knee remained big, black and blue.

I went to school the following morning with a compression band on my knee, which helped it feel better. I was still limping a little, but I THOUGHT I was a lot better. I was called out of class so that my dad and I could go visit our family doctor. He checked it out and said that he didn't think it was anything to worry about and to just keep an eye on it. That was comforting — but it DID NOT get better. The knee remained big, black and blue.

Completely torn

It was time to see a specialist. In order to see a doctor who specialized in busted knees (orthopedist) we had to get approval from our family doctor. After gaining approval and making the appointment we finally met with the new guy. He played with my knee and leg — pushing and pulling — and concluded that something was definitely wrong. He had us go get an MRI to find out for sure what that was.

When I went to get my MRI I was kind of scared. They had me lay down on a stretcher-like thing and slid me into a machine so that only my head stuck out. They clamped earphones on me because the machine made such loud noises. I was in there for a long time. When it was over they said the results would be sent to the doctor.

When we revisited the orthopedist, I was totally unprepared for my diagnosis. He said I had COMPLETELY TORN my ACL and that I would need surgery. Surgery would require taking a piece of my hamstring and using it to replace my ACL. I was devastated.

I never imagined I would ever need surgery. I mean that was pretty crazy. I felt kind of numb. The idea of being cut open frightened me. Not to mention that my injury wasn't a quick fix where I would be back in the game in a couple of weeks. My whole world was suddenly crashing down. There was nothing positive that I could think of to tell myself. Luckily, I had my mom, dad and friends to help me overcome.

> **I never imagined I would ever need surgery. I mean that was pretty crazy.**

After breaking the news, the doctor confessed that he was unable to perform this surgery, but that he knew a doctor who could. I really just wanted to find a doctor who could fix me! He also shared his concern that I might be too young to have the surgical procedure because my bones were still growing. If the surgery went wrong it could stunt my growth. I'm thinking, what does THAT mean? I was at a loss and in the dumps.

We went to see the new doctor and guess

what? He said he was unable to perform the procedure as well. However, he referred us to the doctor that would finally perform my first ACL surgery.

Cut open

After discussing the procedure that would occur during the operation, we set up a date. After setting a date a week away, the whole situation really hit me — I was going to be put to sleep and CUT OPEN. But I was also glad that it was finally going to happen and be over with. There were a bunch of rules that I had to follow the day before, like no eating and drinking after a certain time. We had to be at the hospital at 7 a.m. for check-in. My dad was on a business trip during this time and was unable to come with me, which was odd because he had never missed out on any big events in my life.

I remember dressing in loose clothing and taking a thorough shower the night before because they said that changing would be easier and I did not know when my next shower would be. I'm glad I did since I did not take a proper shower for the next two weeks (I washed up at the bathroom sink). After they took me in, I changed into scrubs and comfy

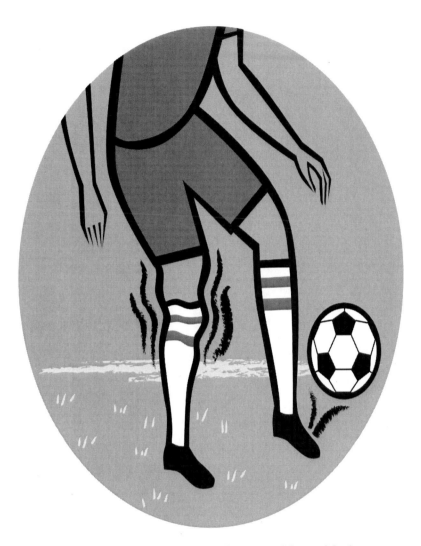

I KNEW that there was a serious problem. My knee was buckling as if it wasn't even connected.

socks. They connected this warm air tube to my robe so that I would stay warm. Next they inserted an IV into my hand. I was glad that my mom was with me. It was a mysterious and forbidding experience.

Mom left and they took me into the operating room. Now THAT was creepy. There were tables with what looked like metallic torture devices and a gurney-like bed with straps. But it was actually quite comfortable once I lay down on it. They inserted anesthesia into my arm and said to count down from five. I don't think I made it past one — I was a goner. I woke in the recovery center confused. One of the nurses explained where I was and that I was all done. I felt drowsy and went in and out of a deep sleep. From my waist down I was numb. I could feel my right leg being weighed down. I checked and, sure enough, I had a massive brace with numerous bandages wrapped around my knee. I went back to sleep.

After reawakening I felt some pain. The nurse gave me a strong pill that worked immediately. Once I was a little more awake I was given some apple juice with a straw. Eventually I was put in a wheelchair and changed. I was still feeling drowsy and fuzzy when I got into the car. I slept the whole way home. I went to my room and pretty much stayed asleep for the next TWO DAYS.

Slowly I started eating a tiny bit and forced myself to drink prune juice. It took some time and effort, but I got the hang of using crutches, going up stairs, bathing, using the bathroom, and other daily activities that I never thought twice about before. After about a week or so, I started attending physical therapy and trying to get my range of

There were tables with what looked like metallic torture devices ...

motion (ROM) back. It was very painful and kind of a slow process. Most of my progress was made at home by continuing my exercises from therapy every day on my own. I went to therapy about twice a week.

Taking a toll

One of the hardest parts about my first torn ACL was going back to school. I had to travel to six classes throughout the day on my crutches and sit in cramped seats. In addition, everyone would look at me or ask me what had happened. It was really uncomfortable because I was so limited in mobility. I had to carry a backpack and I needed friends to help me get from one class to another. During this time period, I sort of went into a mini depression. I felt very alone and useless. I needed assistance for almost everything. It was especially hard because my athletic lifestyle was over. After spending about 75 percent of my life in club soccer, it was strange and difficult to transition to an inactive existence ... which was to last for MONTHS. And I missed my teammates.

The lack of exercise after I had surgery really took a toll on me emotionally.

During my recovery, I spent much of my time reading, which helped me escape from my misery and blue thoughts. In time I was able to take showers again (with a plastic chair in the tub) and discarded my crutches. The brace had to stay on a whole lot longer though. I learned which outfits I could wear and how to recreate my morning routine to prepare for school.

Coming back

After I had finished general therapy, I began specialized sports rehabilitation therapy to make ready for a reentry into athletics. This involved strengthening my leg and core muscles. I gradually started to exercise again. This was VERY GRADUAL. If I overdid it, my knee would shoot with pain the next day. After I stopped attending physical therapy sessions, I continued to do the exercises at home and at my local gym. Rehab took months, but I finally starting to feel like myself again and then some. These exercise programs got me into the best shape of my life.

> I felt very alone and useless. I needed assistance for almost everything.

Returning to school my junior year, I joined the cross-country team. After months of being unable to exercise at all, I had found a new love for running (of course with the years of soccer I wasn't a stranger to that at all). Each day after school our team would take long, hilly runs in the surrounding neighborhoods or spend time on the track working on time. My workout experience was richer now because I had my friends and a team to run with.

The following season I decided to try out for the lacrosse team. I spent a couple of weeks in advance learning the game and practicing. When tryouts came, I almost made varsity, but because it was my first year playing, the coach wanted me to start junior varsity and possibly move up as the season went on. I really enjoyed the game and learning a new sport. My whole life I had only played soccer and because it took so much time, I was never able to really try another sport. I was on a roll — feeling great and getting better every day.

World's end

Then it happened again. During the opening minutes of our second game I had the ball and was trying to escape a defender. One wrong twist and I was on the ground holding my knee. It's INSANE how quickly you can feel at the top of your game one minute and like the world is going to end the next. Even though I was the one who got hurt, I felt as if I had let down the people around me. Especially my dad. When I really realized what had happened I started crying. Yes, my knee hurt, but it wasn't the pain that brought the tears.

When I saw my dad I apologized to him. I don't really know why I did, but I think it was because I knew how hard my surgery and recovery had been for me and my family, and it was going to happen ALL OVER AGAIN.

After a couple of days resting my swollen knee, we were able to get an approval from my family doctor to see a specialist. After confirming my torn ACL and partial meniscus bruising with an MRI, I just wanted to set up a surgery date and get the process moving. The difference this time is that I felt a lot braver — I knew the process and what was going to happen. I knew that I would make it OK and that it was something that I was just going to have to go through again. Complaining and feeling bad for myself would not help me, only make things worse. I just kept telling myself that bad things happen to people and reminding myself of all the things in my life to be grateful for.

I felt like I could live my life and continue through the process STRONG.

Positivity

Positive thinking and embracing the idea that "it is what it is" really helped me this time around. To help with my recovery, I continued to exercise every day until the day of my surgery. The doctor said that the stronger you go into surgery, the faster it is to recover. I think that continuing my exercise routine before surgery kept me positive and determined. I did not feel "handicapped" so to speak. I felt like I could live my life and continue through the process STRONG.

When surgery day finally came around I was nervous, but kind of excited that things were moving along. I thought the sooner I had the surgery, the sooner I could recover. Dad was with me this time.

When I found out for sure that I had torn my ACL again, I immediately rescheduled my summer. Originally, I was going to get a head start on my senior year by taking classes in summer school for the first few weeks of vacation. After that I was signed up to volunteer at an aquatic sports camp as a counselor-in-training for the rest of the break. However, because of the injury, I scheduled my surgery as soon as my vacation started in June. That way I would have most of my break to recover. I was able to take the classes during the second half of my summer.

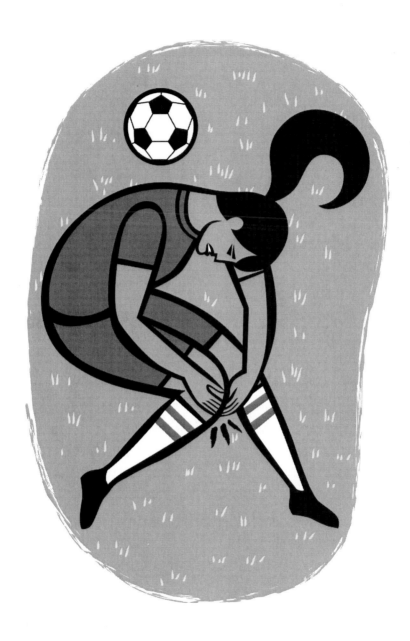

Repeat journey

I trudged into the surgery room in my hospital robe with all the familiar tubes and wires sprouting from me. The doctors and medical assistants were waiting and introduced themselves and asked me to lie down. They inserted the drugs and just like that I was out. Unlike the last time, I didn't even count backwards. When I woke up, I was a little foggy, but awake. Again, it was a very weird feeling not to be able to feel my bottom half. One of the nurses noticed I was awake and asked me how I felt. She returned with some saltine crackers and apple juice. I felt a lot more awake and aware than the first time.

On the way out, the doctor told me to just focus on wiggling my toes to bring feeling back into my legs. I was given two different types of painkillers — one for severe pain and another for lesser pain. We arrived home and I settled on the couch. After my first surgery, I stayed asleep and out of it for a couple of days before I started feeling normal again. This time when I got home I was awake and watching movies.

Over the next month I spent most of my time reading, doing homework and trying out new things. I had mixed feelings of relief — because my surgery was over and I was on the road to recovery — but also frustration because it was summer and here I was stuck inside with my crutches. Fortunately, my family was very thoughtful and helpful. They planned numerous outings that I could participate in. For example, we visited the Wild Animal Park and saw a new exhibit. It worked out perfectly because I was able to see everything and have a good time from a wheel chair.

I conquered my misfortunes one step at a time.

Activities like this really kept my spirits up. My parents' support and motivation were a big help. In addition, I think that because I was ready for all of the changes that would come with recovery, I was able to make sure that my grades and attitude did not slip.

During therapy, I worked hard and was adamant about continuing and pushing myself throughout my exercises. The most difficult part of the recovery process was that even though I was starting to feel better and able to walk, I still had to wear a brace and use crutches. This was very frustrating.

Stronger

I was very happy to start doing short periods of gym work, but perhaps a bit too eager. I pushed too hard one day. At the time it felt fine — like I was just getting a good workout. But the next day I couldn't even walk because my knee hurt so much. Eventually I returned to my gym routine, tuning it to fit my recovery level. I think that by getting back into an exercising routine, even if it was limited because of recovery protocol, I was able to maintain a positive attitude and feel "normal" again.

My overall experience in dealing with my injuries made me a stronger person. After overcoming and moving forward, I often compare current difficulties to that experience. As a rule, today's problems are minor in comparison.

No one plans or expects misfortunes to occur, however when they arrive (and they will arrive), you just have to gather yourself, figure out your next step and then the next step after that. I conquered my misfortunes one step at a time.

2. *First injury*
Dad's notes

I did not see the incident that caused Joy's first ACL injury. Oh, I was there, just not looking up at the time. I was watching, glanced away and when I looked back she was in a heap on the turf clutching her leg. I was told that she had a mild collision with an opposing player, but nothing violent. The game had just started and motors weren't yet on high.

Just ignore it! It'll go away! Now, get after that ball!

Like most parents, especially dads (although moms aren't that far behind), I was impatient with the break in action. *Come on, Joy! Get back up and dominate!* Just before the game started during warmups, one of Joy's teammates went limp with a charlie horse and her dad called out from the stands. *Walk it off, Demi!* This something so many of us parents say, or at least think, when injury first arrives. *Just ignore it! It'll go away! Now, get after that ball!* As I recall, Demi's spasmodic calf settled and she did, in fact, overcome and play up to speed.

But Joy enjoyed no such reprieve, although she gallantly tried to prevail. She left the game and on the sidelines began the walking off process. Soon she was running sprints behind the bench and to my delight re-entered the contest with gusto. *That's my girl!*

The glorious return (and it was glorious — fallen player who picks herself off the pitch, willing her leg to work and dashing back to the fray), was short lived. Joy waved to her coach, pointed to her uncooperative limb and hitched back to the bench. Later she told me that it wasn't pain that compelled her to bow out, but that her leg was wobbly — bending the wrong way (think about *that* for a second — about your lower leg bending not just back, but *forward* and *side-to-side* as well.

I made my way (self-consciously) from the stands to the bench and immediately felt out of place — as I most certainly was. Standing there, patting my daughter on the head while she sat in quiet misery with her cheering teammates. *Sorry daddy*, she said. Someone from the tournament, a sort of first aid person, showed up with a cloth wrap and an ice pack and expertly prepared the first aid on the soon-to-be swollen knee. No more games this weekend. Throughout my daughter was stoic. She told me later she cried a bit, but I did not see it. *I knew it was bad,* she said. *It hurt and I cried, and I never cry.*

I left her on the bench and went back to the stands and *that* felt strange. Leaving my injured child so she could remain with her team on the bench and I could sit with the other parents and pretend that I gave a hoot about the game. That's the sporting way, I guess. I mean, if I can't wave a magic wand and cure the knee and get Joy back into game and glory, I don't want to be there. The truth is, if my daughter isn't playing, I don't care about anything else. Don't get me wrong — I grew to love the parents and their kids. They were my life outside of my family. But as far as the playing and the coaching, if Joy isn't on the field, I'm not on the sidelines. I am 100 percent my daughter's doting dad and there is not much left over for team spirit or for the love of the game.

I knew it was bad, she said. It hurt and I cried, and I never cry.

After the game I talked to the first aid tent and the coach and anyone else who wanted to talk to me about banged up knees. *So what is the problem? She needs to see a doctor. Maybe it's just a sprain. Maybe it's just the meniscus. What's the meniscus? Something that will heal without a fuss. Keep it up. Keep it iced.* Meanwhile the knee is getting bigger and redder. It does not look like anything minor or anything asking to be merely walked off. But who knows.

Better go see a doctor.

Finding a doctor

There was one parent who knew what was coming. We were sitting in the hotel lobby the next morning waiting to congregate and ship out. One of the dads said, *So you gonna get an MRI?* I said, *We'll see a doctor all right* and pretty much left it at that. I didn't know what an MRI was exactly and part of me was still very much thinking this was a self-healing sort of thing. I knew MRIs were connected to serious sporting activity. Football players had MRIs. Baseball pitchers had MRIs. But kids got sprains, right? *Hey, just walk it off!*

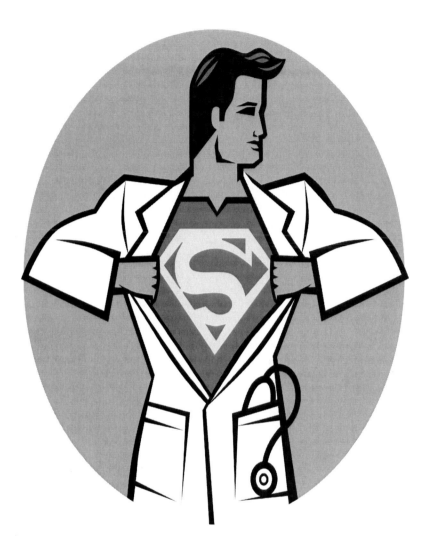

Some of these people are racehorses — thorough-breds who live for the surgical event and the miracle of reconstruction. And that's a good thing. You want your surgeon to be talented and ever so confident — no doubt about that.

Our first doctor visits didn't clear anything up. Unfortunately, our family physician didn't know a thing about bones or ligaments in general or knees in particular. He pulled and twisted Joy's right lower leg a bit (which was hard to watch) and didn't discover anything to report. *Give it some time and we'll see.* Which, of course, fed the hopeful man inside who was looking for the easy fix. *So when can she play, doc?*

After some time nothing got better and we thought it best to find a bone doctor (orthopedist). Our insurance required that our primary physician OK that and so I camped out at the office, corralled one of the nurses to help me and got a referral to see one. *The doctor knows him very well. He's been around for a very long time.* And in time that proved to be a problem because this fellow was older, not so much working with athletes anymore and disinclined to work with us.

But he did order an MRI. And that was the beginning of the beginning. Before the MRI, you're guessing. Everybody's guessing. It's the MRI that tells the truth. There is something else that our second orthopedist used, a sort of flex-o-meter — a mechanical device that measures a ligament's range of motion, but even after that we went for the MRI to really see inside the knee.

So Joy and I go to the imaging facility that houses the large contraption that provides MRIs and for the first time in her young life, she goes to see a medical professional without mom or dad. The MRI guy actually laughed when I started to walk into the room with her. *We can't have you in there. Just Joy.* A mild shock. They do grow up.

But kids got sprains, right? *Hey, just walk it off!*

So it's been a few weeks since the injury occurred. Waited some time to see the first doc. Waited some more time after the first visit. Waited a bit to get an appointment with the second doc and we had to wait to get the MRI. Finally, we had to wait for the results.

They don't just call you up with the results. You have to make an appointment, wait outside the door, wait inside one of the little rooms and wait for someone to stop by and tell you the news. Which, in this case, was like the earth lurching on its axis. Because it was very bad news, indeed. Joy's ACL was completely torn in two. Snapped.

The hopeful little man inside was squashed. Brutally vanquished. I remember the doctor's assistant giving me the report along with a simple guide to ligaments and ligament injury. *Oh man. Really?* The orthopedist finally appeared and said he no longer did the surgery, but that a neighboring orthopedist did and referred us to him. We made an appointment for the next week and ... waited.

Joy, as is her style, was composed. She didn't cry or say anything. I think she is tough in the finest way a person can be. Some get to be tough only through anger or meanness. Like you need a shot of nastiness to forge ahead. I know I can be like that. But I think Joy is just strong. Strong enough within herself to take it. Not that she wasn't affected by the grim results. She got quiet and I knew it hurt. Of course it did.

So we see the new guy in a week or so and he tells us that he specializes in hips, not knees. But he will help us find the right guy. This, of course, is getting laughable. It's been weeks since she's been hurt and we're still fiddling with who's gonna be our doc and what he's gonna do. It took one MD to see another, who got us an MRI, who sent us to another MD who will send us off to see yet another MD. If you're scoring, that's MDa to MDb to MRI to MDc to MDd.

> Joy, as is her style, was composed. I think she is tough in the finest way a person can be.

Out of all that, the only thing truly of worth was the MRI that tells it like it is. It sees the ligaments and registers the damaged tissue as well as an x-ray sees the broken bones. The experience taught me the value of MRIs and the importance of getting one after a knee injury as soon as possible.

To be fair, one of the doctors did review x-rays and OK'd Joy for the surgery which is an iffy thing in children and a crucial decision to make. Fool around with bone and ligament too early, and the kid will not develop properly. If Joy had not been ready for an operation, we would have had to wait for physical maturation.

Clueless

Looking back, I can see how unreasonably optimistic we were (or I was) about the extent of the knee damage. In the *weeks* it took to finally get the MRI, which dispelled all hope for a quick fix, Joy signed up for another year with her soccer club team and another summer as a counselor-in-training (CIT) at her sailing camp.

I remember her refereeing a soccer scrimmage one evening. Coaches knew she had hurt her leg, but thought just limping through ref duty would be light enough work and still get her into the swim of things (it makes sense if you're a part of this scene). So she's out there with all these charging young ladies (and by this age their charging has become quite formidable), dragging her bum leg and faking a take at officiating. This did not last long.

To my credit, as the responsible parent I can be at times, I put the kibosh on this when I showed up at practice. This is sort of a medium-sized deal, by the way. dads just don't interfere in club soccer practice or games, as all obedient club soccer parents know — and make no mistake — I was an obedient parent for many years. But upon seeing my daughter wobbling out there among her thundering teammates, I reflexively took action and (boldly!) took her out of the game. I'm not proud of most of my sideline antics over the course of Joy's soccer career, but I feel OK about this one.

Summer camp was a joke. She showed up each morning and lumbered about helping with those things less physical. Meaning she didn't work with boats, which was pretty much what she was there for. This and soccer went up in smoke after the MRI, of course. To their credit, both the soccer club* and sailing center returned the monies spent.

It's been weeks ... and we're still fiddling with who's gonna be our doc.

So I guess you could say we resided somewhere between not knowing and denial. I sorta heard the rumbling, but the stampeding truth was just over the hill and out of sight.

Meanwhile she was *on the leg*. Walking around, going places, doing things. Her leg unstable

*I gotta say, though, that Joy's head coach never said a thing. No good-bye, no get well soon, no wishing you the best. Unconscionable. The lack of regard is stunning if you consider the relationships involved in the world of club soccer.

because the most important ligament in her right knee had burst asunder. But the swelling had gone down and it *looked better. Gee, maybe it'll be OK.*

Not buying it

There is an undercurrent of disbelief among coaches and parents and players when you first deal with injury. It's a belief married to the *Just walk it off* mentality — like you're faking it. Or you lack resolve. As if a player should simply be able to *will* the injury away.

When Joy went back to school after surgery all braced up with crutches, she had to deal with a coach who thought along these lines. This fellow taught a gym class that Joy was in and grew skeptical when her knee did not heal according to his timeline. *I had a sprain and I was back in six weeks. Never heard of a sprain taking so long to heal.* So he gave her a middling grade when she couldn't do sprints. Fortunately, Joy's guidance counselor was a former high school and college athlete who had suffered *six(!)* knee operations in her career. She caught wind of the grade and educated coach to a more enlightened state.

That I would have paid to see.

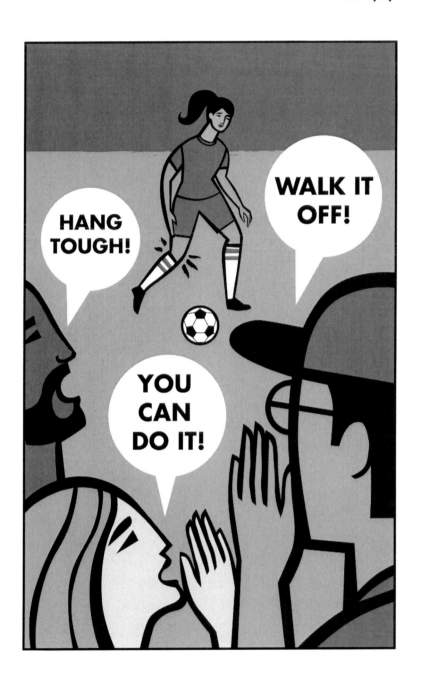

Finally

To his credit, the last of our do-little MDs found us *the* guy — the doctor who would mend the knee for real. Remember the fellow who urged his daughter Demi to walk off her calf spasm? Happened he was a medical technician who knew a little something about this doctor and did us the kindness of checking him out. *He's all right. You're in good hands.* This good turn, by the way, is an indication of the family feel I still miss with the club soccer business. These folks were my best friends for about three years.

His office (he shared with other doctors) was impressively hung with photos of name athletes thanking various orthopedists for fixing them up. San Diego, after all, is a pretty big city and a sports mecca to boot, so this came as no surprise. The staff was very professional. Signing us in, guiding us to a room, asking questions, filling out forms, prepping us for the orthopedist who showed after a short while.

The doctor was pleasant and calm. Knew his stuff. Had done a lot of these surgeries. He explained what he was going to do. It felt like our ship had finally come in. We were hoping for an operation date that would not interfere too much with school and, as luck would have it, there was an opening sooner than expected. For the first time in all this, our journey was expedited.

Joy was hurt in April. She finally got surgery in July.

A long day

It's a belief married to the *Just walk it off* mentality — like you're faking it.

I was in Tennessee on business the day Joy had surgery. Her mother took her in for the out-patient procedure that took most of the morning. She was prepped and carted away while Kathleen hung out in the waiting room, checking out Joy's progress on a monitor installed there. The screen updated each step as it occurred and lent a little light to an experience that would otherwise have felt pretty mysterious.

As it was, my wife and I were a bit anxious since this was the first operation any of us ever had to endure. Once Kathleen was run over by a bicyclist and bumped her head, but nothing cracked. I've had cuts, sprains and broken fingers, but nothing very serious. Joy was the first to go under and get cut open. I took *that* very seriously.

Being 2,000 miles away did not help. Kathleen and I traded texts which seemed better than talking for some reason. We are both literal communicators and discussing the morning's proceedings via the written word was the way to go. Anyway, I remember that 3-4 hour span of time as being intensely emotional — about as emotional as anything I ever felt.

Physical therapy

For several weeks Joy underwent physical therapy or PT. The first few weeks she worked with what I'd call a general therapist who got her to slowly regain flexibility and strength. These were 45 minute sessions, twice a week.

After about six weeks or so, Joy switched to a PT program designed for athletes. Joy wanted to resume an athletic interest of some sort, and we were told by doctors and coaches that a more intensive PT was required to build the kind of muscle and sturdiness around her injured knee that such exertion demands. Especially in those sports that require pivoting and explosive changes in direction like soccer or lacrosse (the latter was of budding interest to Joy).

The folks at what I'll call the sport therapy center were, in fact, athletes (the guy we initially used was not) and really worked Joy hard. Again, these were 45 to 60 minute sessions and our girl dearly felt the hard work. In short order, Joy began to lose the softness that had set in after her injury and gradually regained tone and then some. Along with that she gained a spring in her step, and I mean that literally as well as figuratively. I would say that by the end of her time with the sport therapy center Joy was in the best shape of her life. Along with that she assumed a vibrant and fresh outlook.

Joy was the first to go under and get cut open. I took *that* very seriously.

The sessions with the sport therapy center came in two parts. Insurance covered bouts for the first few weeks. These got Joy a dedicated therapist one-on-one and it's here that she made the greatest strides. Like I said, these young people were athletes. Joy worked with a

competitive female weightlifter, college soccer
players and a triathlete. They were the real deal
and brooked no gutless effort. You gave them
(and yourself, of course) your best shot for the
entire 45 minutes. However, it must be said that
their seriousness did not include harshness. It
wasn't like a boot camp with a lot of hollering
and browbeating. I would call it more like an
enthusiastic intensity based on good intentions.
*We will make you better! And stronger! And
more confident! We will get you back in the
game!*

And they did.

When the insurance ran out, we signed on for
group classes (I say *we* because I took them
with Joy). These were economically priced, get-
fit sessions that emphasized core muscle work
led by one of the therapists, but usually
included a couple of the others who wanted to
tag along. It was a fun bunch of six to eight
clients plus a therapist or two and, like the one-
on-ones, the sessions required much effort. I
was usually drenched after class and sore the
next day. The switch to classes did not impede
Joy's progress at all. It was the same therapy,
just spread out a little. It also gave me something so very worthwhile to do with my

daughter, and this was not a small thing for either one of us.

The only drawback, the only one, was travel time. It took maybe 25 minutes or so to get to the center. Sometimes the sessions ran a little late into the evening for a school night, thus yielding a longish day. But this is almost niggling to complain about since the benefits of working with the program were whopping.

We will get you back in the game!

And they did.

Back in the saddle

Joy was in the waning weeks of her sophomore year in high school when she was pronounced fit to compete. Joy jumped back into the sporting life with cross-country. It felt like a minor miracle to hear her tell of long runs with teammates up and over hills and fields.

The leg was working again!

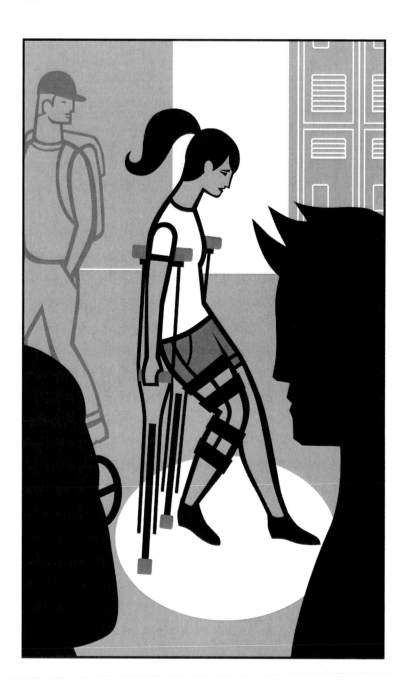

3. *Once more*
Dad's notes

Again

After her cross-country stint, Joy really wanted to play lacrosse. Since she had never played, she asked her friends on the lacrosse team to help her learn so she could try out come Spring. She buttonholed players to teach her after school and weekends and even got me to lend a hand. On her own, she'd walk around cradling the ball in the house and yard.

> Most times I (and we) just shrug it off and are content to deal with the setback.

I've got to hand it to her how she endeavored to learn and work so hard to gain proficiency. I think of that sometimes and get a stab of pain, about the only time I feel sorry or pity about how things worked out for my daughter. Most times I (and we) just shrug it off and are content to deal with the setback. Looking ahead seems easier this time than the first. Like, OK, we've been here before and know what to do. No need to complain. But remembering how she made herself into a player — how happy and proud she was to make the team — it still hurts.

Pop!

It was the last thing on my mind, Joy getting hurt again. After 12 months of repair and rehab I thought her knee was as good as new. She was strong and fit — in absolutely tip-top condition.

The lacrosse game was about ten minutes old, Joy playing forward in her second game (ever). I was standing on the top level of seats so I could take it all in. She could see me easily. Before the whistle Joy looked up and we waved at each other.

Of course I got excited each time she touched the ball and there were a few times that happened. Play was sloppy and awkward, (after all, this was JV), but who cared? There was Joy, rambling with her stick on the field of play. *Back in the game!*

The ball gets tossed back and forth, here and there during a lacrosse match. Since the girls are new at the game, much of the time it doesn't go where intended or caught so there's some scrambling and knots of energetic players converging with scooping sticks. From up top it looked fairly tame. Nothing violent. Just exuberant.

It was during one of these mashups that Joy went down clutching her knee. Yes, that knee. She stayed down and on some level I knew it was serious, although the mind immediately countered with the usual *Maybe it's OK* thought pattern —

> There was Joy, rambling with her stick on the field of play. *Back in the game!*

a sort of trick to keep a parent's worried mind from exploding, I guess.

What was I feeling then? Deflation. Numbness. Acquiescence.

Like the first time, I sheepishly clambered down the stadium steps and approached the bench where my daughter sat with an ice wrap. I stopped at the fence barrier a few feet away, not wanting to disturb the sanctity of bench and team and wondered if that was appropriate. Joy may have looked up, I don't remember. I knew she was hurting and miserable. Coach talked to her a bit. Other players, too.

I finally made a quick visit to the bench.

I heard it pop, daddy. I'm sorry.

Her saying that raised some eyebrows among her team, but she didn't mean it as an apology to me — that she had failed her father. I think she meant it as an expression of sorrow that such an awful thing could have happened to her again. Anyway, it was the "pop" that defined the moment. All the physical examinations and scanning to come was just procedure and grim confirmation of what that pop indicated. A pop does not say slight sprain. It says a ligament has been snapped, thank you very much, and that for the next nine months of your life you will be struggling to heal. Or in our case, to reheal.

I went back to the fence and stood there behind the team with the crowd behind my back and waited for the game to end. Haplessly. Almost foolishly. What on earth is a parent supposed to do when his kid gets hurt? Run on to the field? Just trust in the coaches and officials and first aid people and wait it out? Is there protocol? *It's awkward, man. Unbelievably awkward.*

The game ended and we trudged to the car and drove home. Joy plunked down on the couch, put her leg up and I prepared the cold compress. I think it was a bag of frozen peas. Maybe blueberries (berries, by the way, can be a problem because when they thaw, they run red and stain). We sat there in a stew of pity, watched TV and waited for mom to come home. I don't remember us having much to say.

Anyway, it was the "pop" that defined the moment.

Kathleen walked through the door all upbeat and smiley like she usually is after a day of meetings and cubicle politics, but was stopped by the air of doom. *What's wrong?*

One of us said, *The knee is hurt again.*

The same knee?

Yes.

Oh, no! You guys seem awfully calm considering.

Calm? Mostly stunned, I'd say.

And stunned I stayed throughout until the MRI results came back, and then I felt like crying.

Special friends

The day Joy went back to school after the ACL was very important and the goodwill she received from a special friend invaluable. Going back in brace, on crutches (again) was a physical and emotional hardship for my daughter. It was tough to get around and difficult to cross campus and get to class on time. It was tough to answer the questions and be stared at. It was really tough to think this was only the beginning of a nine-month process. Much reason to be depressed — and she was.

There was a pivotal moment when the advance of Joy's depression was blocked, averted and replaced with hope and determination.

The second injury occurred early on during her Spring break. She had a week or so at home before school started up again and much of that time was spent stewing in bed or on the couch. Of course, Kathleen and I (with our dog Blue) consoled, provided and pampered as best we could, but still we are *family* — fundamental, but not an entirely complete support system.

> She had to go back to that other universe — high school — on a pair of crutches.

She had to go back to that other universe — high school — on a pair of crutches. Back to a campus full of friends, teammates, acquaintances, teachers and classrooms. All eyes upon her. Limping between classes, trying to keep up with the surging flow. Just sitting down in a chair and getting up with cast and crutches such a supreme hassle. She was an invalid, at least for the time being. A person apart.

Her best friend knew what to do. On her first day back, he took her to see the same counselor who had stood up to the ignorant gym teacher several months ago who was suspicious of Joy's first knee injury. This was the person, who as a student athlete, had had six knee operations.

Meeting with such a valued and respected adult friend and advisor *who had been there before* was exactly what Joy needed at exactly the correct time. It bucked Joy up and helped set the tone for her healing and recovery. I was not in the room, but I'm sure it was one of those special times, probably just a few minutes long, where a connection was made and a course set that made all the difference. Two good friends made the effort and I am forever grateful for their intelligent and generous response.

Simpler

After that it was an unremarkable emotional journey this time. Putting one foot in front of the other and notching each step in the healing process.

It was a great settling of matters for me. And probably for Joy, too. The second injury meant an end to high school and club sports. No more tryouts, no more practice, no more games, no more time away from studies and family. Unlike the first blown knee, there was no pressure to get well and get back to the team. This was the

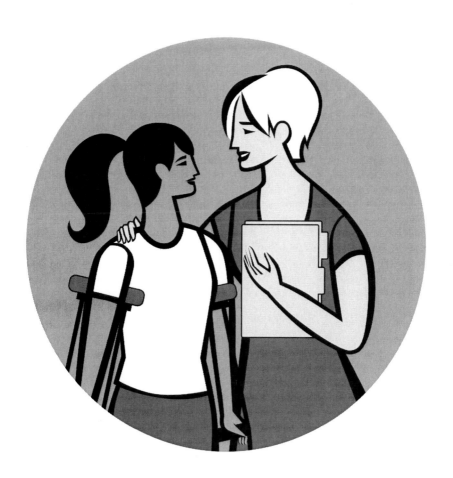

end. All at once life was a lot simpler.

Sure there was some missing out. Being a part of a team. Being active. Striving to win and to play your best. But Joy had been an athlete for several years at this point. Her resume included club soccer, high school cross-country, soccer and lacrosse and sailing and other water sports at an aquatic center each summer. She had had more than a taste of the sporting life. Quite frankly, her athletic activities sometimes overwhelmed our lives.

As things turned out, she had more time to study and to participate in other activities like drama and her other clubs at school. It was OK. Really. It was even a *relief.*

Not that I let go right away.

Final word

At first I pursued the thought that maybe it was not the ACL, that the injury was something less serious. Remembering the frittering of time after the first ACL tear, I asked our primary care physician to OK a visit to a specialist as soon as possible. He asked if I wanted him to check her out first, but I said I pretty much knew that the next step was the bone doctor.

I was abrupt — very keen on getting an MRI and you need an orthopedic doctor to sign off on that. Looking back I may have been unkind, although I didn't mean to be. I wanted to know for certain what happened inside of Joy's knee. And I wanted to know ASAP. To his credit, he overlooked my impatience and OK'd the visit to the orthopedic doc.

> **Quite frankly, her athletic activities sometimes overwhelmed our lives.**

A strong positive was that the new doctor was very close by — about a half mile from our house. I had met him before. Years ago I broke a pinkie and he looked it over. What I remember is that I did not have insurance at the time and he gave me a break on the visit. Good guy.

The bad news was the result of the physical exam. One of the doctors (there were two that we dealt with, the main guy I mentioned before and a second in charge) did a hands-on inspection of Joy's knee and followed that with another that utilized a contraption that strapped on the leg and measured laxity as it emitted sharp popping noises. The knee was so loose that they did the test a few times just to make sure they got it right. We were sent off to get an MRI, but it was pretty clear that doctors and staff all thought the ligament was toast.

Sure enough, the results came back showing that the ACL was once again ripped apart. There were brief thoughts that maybe the first surgery wasn't done properly. I mean, wasn't it supposed to be good as new? Strong as ever? But our new doctor said he didn't think so, although he'd know more when he got in there. I got the feeling that he thought that the rerupturing of the knee was just one of those things, not malpractice. We didn't seriously entertain that it was. The first guy had a great rep, the knee rehabbed well and stood up to a season of cross-country and a preseason of lacrosse. It was another bad piece of luck. And probably a case of predisposition. The hard truth (I have come to think) is that Joy's knees are simply too loose for cutting sports.

After that visit I remember taking Joy to school, filling in the attendance clerk about her absence and walking back to the car with a welling in my chest. Joy had been stoic, more bummed then sorrowful about facing another bout with brace and crutches. But I felt so sad about her dashed ambitions to play high school sports and so angry that she had to deal with another reconstruction. *The injustice of it all!* I felt like shaking my fist ... at who? God? The fates? It was my lowest moment.

However, it did not last long. What took over was a sense of *practicality*. A patient desire to get on with it.

Maybe she has to modify her ambitions, but that's OK. *Life goes on.*

That's what we did and that's what's getting us through. The thing is, it may be rotten when it happens, but the body does heal. It does get better. It's not like losing a limb or getting an incurable disease. The player gets patched up and heals. Maybe to go back out on the field or maybe not. Maybe she has to modify her ambitions, but that's OK. This life presents all sorts of things to do. Any number of pursuits are out there to kindle interest and passion.

Life goes on.

Another surgery

This time it was my turn to take Joy to the surgeon. Unlike the facility where the first surgery was performed, this hospital was only about 10 minutes away. We got there with time to spare. But like everything else medical, you show up and wait. Go to the next thing and wait. And so on and so forth.

After check-in we went to a tiny room to get prepped. Joy was upbeat, not nervous. I sat with her until the doctor was ready to roll, then sat in the waiting area until she was done. There was a screen in the room indicating the progress of each patient scheduled to receive treatment that day.

I saw (via the screen) Joy go through her sequence of surgical events and after a couple of hours a nurse came out to tell me how great the surgery went and how great our surgeon was and how she'd seen him work miracles with cases so much worse than ours. And this was great to hear, of course. *Exactly* what a parent wants to hear, in fact, after their child goes through this sort of thing.

The doctor came out to brief me on the surgery and in short to tell me all went well.

This fellow really appeared to know his stuff and I appreciated his follow up. He showed me images taken from the tiny camera that he had poked about in her knee. Although it was hard to know what I was looking at, it's mighty impressive that this point of view is available — that we can see inside the joint, under the skin and tissue without a ghastly excavation as was required not so very long ago. Arthroscopic surgery is indeed a technological marvel.

Arthroscopic surgery is indeed a technological marvel.

I asked if he had an opinion of the first surgery after looking around in there and he said there was no indication that the first reconstruction wasn't up to snuff. Part of me thinks *What else is he going to say? Do you really think he'd indict a fellow MD?* But maybe that's being a bit cynical. I remember him saying *Every injury is different, every surgery is different.* And that's what I took away from that turn in the conversation.

I thanked him and told him how much the nurse thought of his performance as a surgeon.

He smiled and said he worked with very good people and that sounded right to me. You watch for the arrogance with these guys and when it's not there it's a pleasant and reassuring thing.

After that I went through the wrong door and set off an alarm that attracted a few medical folks who patiently and kindly pointed me in the right direction. What's a trip to the hospital without getting lost?

In a bit they wheeled Joy and her braced leg out, she piled into the van I had brought around and off we went. Joy said that they didn't drug her up as much as last time and, as a result, felt better than before.

When we got home she propped herself on the couch and conked out. Thus began the healing process that would take ... so ... much ... time.

CPM

Initial rehab for the repaired knee involves re-establishing and improving range of motion. This can be done with professional physical therapy or a device called a continuous passive motion (CPM) machine. After her first ACL

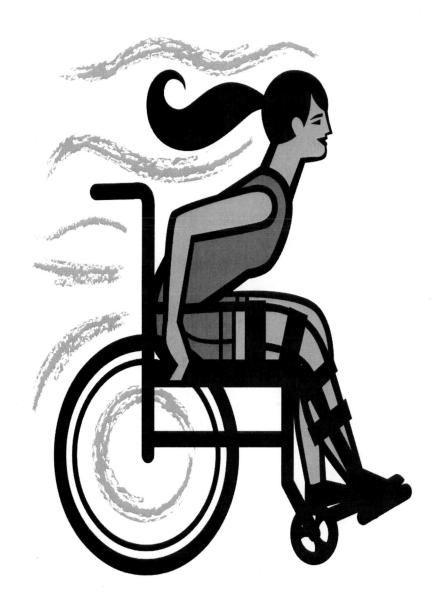

surgery Joy did simple exercises prescribed by a physical therapist. This time we got a machine.

The thing was strapped to Joy's leg and gradually bent it to a prescribed point while she was lying back on the couch. The machine had a setting that could be adjusted to allow for more acute bending as the knee mended. Slowly — very slowly — the machine angled her leg and straightened it out again. Over and over and over. Joy could study or read or watch TV while this was going on without giving it a thought. It was convenient, effective and easy.

Wheeling around

Joy and I were intent on getting on with things and moving around. Laying about was so easy to do with the injury — putting off exercising, errands and more important projects. I got the idea of wheelchair workouts when we decided to visit some colleges over Spring break. She obviously couldn't walk around very well so we rented a chair for the week and tooled around Cal State Long Beach, USC, Cal State Northridge and UC Santa Barbara (where she ended up going).

Without thinking, I did most of the powering at

first, but it eventually dawned on me that if I got Joy to roll the thing she'd get some exercise. It was hard to steer since her leg was held up and out in its brace, thus causing an imbalance. I lent a guiding hand with which she was able to motor along by pushing the wheels herself. It proved to be a terrific workout for arms and shoulders and when she really rocked, I'm sure she got her core involved as well.

Look at her go! That bum leg isn't slowing her down!

In time we developed interval training sessions that we executed every other day. Usually trading a count of 10 at a walking pace with a 10-count going full bore. We'd do that for about two miles. It was a great upper body exercise that utilized a significant swath of muscle and dealt a bit of a burn. This was not exactly an aerobic blast, but it did get the heart rate up, burned some calories and got her moving in a serious way. It was work, good work, that was beneficial for head and heart. And one more thing: racing around in a wheelchair turns heads and brings smiles — *Look at her go! That bum leg isn't slowing her down!*

Everyday appreciation for the kid zooming around in a wheelchair.

Worked for her.

Throwing them away!
One hundred and ten days after Joy's second ACL surgery, the doctor took off the brace. One hundred and ten days of recuperation, crutches, straps and struts were over. With considerable care, she could navigate this world without artificial support. When she looked in the mirror she could see both legs. When she walked to and from her high school classes, she looked like everyone else.

No, she could not run or cut or jump. But Joy could walk and use the stationary bike. It wasn't even the beginning of the end. Full recovery was at least another four months away. But at this moment she began to hold herself up all by herself and that was cause for celebration.

It was a fine day.

4. ACL overview
About the great stabilizer

The anterior cruciate ligament (better known as the ACL) is one of four major ligaments in the knee. Ligaments are tissues that connect one bone to another. In a mature knee, the ACL prevents the tibia from moving forward and provides a whopping 90 percent of the knee's stability. The tibia is the larger and stronger of the two lower leg bones connecting knee and ankle.

What an ACL does is ALOT:

1. Keeps the tibia (larger lower leg bone) from moving forward, away from the femur (upper leg bone).

2. Limits excessive knee extension (lower leg bends forward, away from back of thigh).

3. Restricts varus (bowleggedness) and valgus (knock kneed) knee displacement.

4. Controls tibial rotation.

5. Protects the menisci (cushioning cartilage between upper and lower leg bones) from damage when a player jumps, cuts and pivots.

Hurt numbers

It is reported that up to 300,000 ACL injuries occur each year in the United States and that about 100,000 are reconstructed. That is, the damaged ligament is surgically replaced. Seventy percent happen during agility sports such as basketball, soccer, skiing and football. Up to eighty percent occur without contact.

Most of the injured are between the ages of 15 and 45 years of age and lead an active life that usually includes sports participation. Males suffer more ACL injuries than females, because there are more male athletes than female. But females have a much greater risk of being injured.

ACL injury rates increase at ages 12 to 13 for girls and they are four to six times more likely to tear an ACL than boys. This injury rate peaks in the teen years and declines in adulthood. Female athletes 15 to 19 years of age represent that portion of the population with the greatest number of injuries.

Trick knee
There was a time when the function of the ACL was little understood. An ACL injury was called a trick knee because it gave out in an unpredictable manner. Sometimes it worked and sometimes it did not.

Consequences of ACL injury

1. Discomfort and disability associated with treatment and up to nine months of rehab.

2. Several thousands of dollars in treatment costs.

3. Poor academic performance if surgery is done during school year (nonholiday).

4. Sport participation may be limited or eliminated. The sporting life is associated with self-esteem, academic success, improved bone health and lower rates of obesity, diabetes, depression and teen pregnancy.

5. Ten times more likely than noninjured to develop early-onset degenerative knee osteoarthritis. That is, they have a greater risk of suffering chronic pain and limitations from knee osteoarthritis by their 20s and 30s. Osteoarthritis is the most common form of arthritis in the knee.The cartilage wears away thus eliminating the cushion between bones. Bone rubs on bone causing pain and bone spurs (build up of bone in areas of bone-on-bone friction).

You are at risk if these factors are present

● Ill-fitting shoes and irregular turf conditions.

● Increased weight and body mass.

● Ligamentios laxity (loose ligaments).

● Subtalar overpronation (feet that roll inwardly).

● Previous ACL injury (risk is 15 times greater than noninjured).

● Female sex (just being a girl is a risk factor as we shall see).

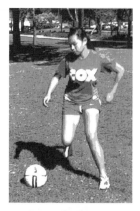

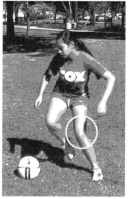

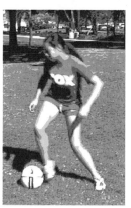

Classic ACL tear

A typical ACL injury happens without contact and involves a fast moving body making or attempting to make a sudden change in direction or speed. These actions include sudden stops, twists or jumps. Cutting is the classic — planting a foot to steer a new course while going full bore. Often the athlete will hear or feel the knee POP! as the ligament breaks. She may continue to play, but the leg will feel wobbly and confidence to execute basic athletic movements will vanish.

An ACL injury can also occur with direct contact on the outside of the knee. Football players, of course, are always crashing into legs. But there's a danger in any sport where players are flying about.

Is it an ACL tear or not?

What the patient knows

Besides hearing the pop during the injury event and having a wobbly leg thereafter, the player may complain of her knee giving out. Pivoting on the offended knee is definitely out. The knee may feel funny — locking up or catching. These are strong indicators of a torn ACL.

Physical examination

There are ways to physically examine the knee, and a doctor trained to do so can accurately determine if the ACL is torn. These examinations involve flexing and applying some kind of force by hand to determine laxity (how much give there is in the knee). If there's too much give, the ligament is damaged.

Validity of physical examination

Although we are trained to think an athletic mishap automatically needs an MRI (magnetic resonance imaging) to determine the extent of injury, physical examination by an expert is sufficient. For example, the Lachman's Test has the doctor pull the tibia (of the injured leg) forward with one hand while holding the thigh just above the knee with the other. If the tibia stays put, the ACL is not torn. If the tibia is pulled forward, the ligament is, in fact, torn. An MRI will confirm the examination and provide some detail.

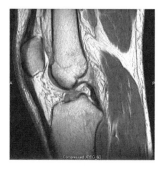

Imaging
An MRI is taken to confirm the finding. Like an x-ray shows the broken bone on a screen for all to see, an MRI provides a picture of the torn ligament. It's the final proof.

No surgery

One does not need to surgically repair the ligament if athletic participation is zero and life after the injury is sedate. Strengthening surrounding muscles and wearing a brace *may* be enough to ward off complications from having an ACL-less appendage.

No surgery is OK, if ...
One of the goals of any treatment is to never let the knee go out of place again. Without an ACL, the knee will buckle under certain stresses and damage cartilage. Cartilage acts as a buffer and shock absorber between upper

and lower leg bones. Losing cartilage can lead to arthritis. If the patient wears a brace and gives up physical activities that require a healthy ACL, like cutting sports, then the main goal of treatment is accomplished.

Surgery

For everyone else, it's reconstruction. Procedure at this time requires a graft, either from the patient or a cadaver.

The repair is done arthroscopically. Small cuts are made to allow a small camera and light inside the knee. What's inside is projected onto a screen so the surgeon can perform surgery through small incision points around the knee. Grafts may come from the patient's patellar, hamstring or quadriceps tendon or, as previously stated, a cadaver.

Replacing the damaged ligament is the way to go. ACLs do not heal and cannot hold a stitch. Says Tarek O. Souryal, M.D., Assistant Clinical Professor, University of Texas Southwestern Medical Center, "The ACL never has the opportunity to mend due to its position and role in the knee — it's very much like a rubber band. That's why this is a forever kind of injury."

Early attempts to repair ACLs this way were failures — an athletic career ended with an ACL injury.

Surgeons began substituting tissue from the patient's patellar tendon, which is located in front of the ACL. But reconstruction before arthroscopic surgery was only a bit more successful. Surgery required that large incisions be made to the knee in order to access the tunnel in which the ligament substitute must reside. Where to place the new tissue was guesswork and the results were usually poor.

It's a far more exact procedure now. With arthroscopic surgery the substitute tissue can be placed precisely where it needs to be. The surgery together with appropriate post-operation physical therapy usually results in a return to sports.

What to expect

ACL reconstruction surgery has a 90 percent success rate regarding knee stability, patient satisfaction and return to full activity. Reconstruction protects parts of the knee from further injury and slows degenerative changes in the knee joint.

> **Damage to other areas of the knee**
> About half of all injuries to the ACL occur along with damage to other structures in the knee, such as the articular cartilage, the meniscus and other ligaments.

There is some debate regarding the chances of re-rupturing the reconstructed knee. Some say there's little chance, some say there's a pretty big chance (see the next subheading).

For those opting out of surgery, there is risk that the knee will suffer further injury and be prone to osteoarthritis.

You want to play again

It has been reported that an athlete who has already suffered an ACL injury is 15 times more likely to get an ACL injury than a previously uninjured athlete.

Research by Mark V. Paterno, PhD, PT, SCS, ATC, and colleagues shows that the risk remains after a year. Over two years, the previously injured player is six times more likely to have another ACL injury — on the same or the opposite knee.

Furthermore, 20 percent of young athletes who returned to sports that require pivoting and cutting movements after ACL surgery experienced a second injury to the opposite leg within two years.

"In our study, female athletes demonstrated more than four times greater rate of injury within twenty-four months after ACL reconstruction than their healthy counterparts. These data highlight the fact that patients who have undergone ACL reconstruction and return to playing sports are at greater risk for injury and should take appropriate precautions to prevent injury," said Dr. Paterno.

Conclusions: Good luck!
Young people who have had ACL reconstruction are at high risk for receiving a second ACL injury — in the same or the opposite knee — up to two years after surgery. This same source reports that females are more than twice as likely to experience an injury to the opposite knee than male athletes.

It is no surprise that this study says current rehabilitation and return to sport protocols need to be reviewed.

Note regarding operating on younger children
Surgery for children younger than 14 years is risky. There is a possibility of arresting normal bone growth that can result in one leg being shorter than the other.

5. *Girls & ACLs*
A special problem

Very strong arguments are being made that female athletes need different strength and conditioning programs than men — that females are predisposed to certain musculoskeletal injuries and medical conditions. Exhibit A for this argument is the very high incidence of ACL injuries among female athletes.

Anatomical differences
Narrow femoral notch
This is the notch in the bone in which the ACL resides. In females this is a narrow, A-shaped notch that may cause a sheering force to the ligament.

Increased Q-angle
Women have wider hips than men that cause the femur to attach to the knee at a greater angle. This stresses the knee and the ACL.

Hormonal differences
There is a thought that the increase in estrogen during menstruation can cause laxity in the ligaments around the knee. It must be said that there is no consensus in the scientific commu-

nity regarding this theory.

However, a want of a certain hormone may be of considerable significance. During puberty's growth spurt, girls experience only a small increase in testosterone, a hormone that helps to control surging body dimensions in boys. Thus this lack of testosterone in pubescent girls prevents the growth of muscle mass and strength required to control fast-growing bodies (longer arms and legs, changing center of mass) during athletic moves.

Flexibility differences

Women are more flexible than men. Hamstring flexibility lessens the ability of these muscles to protect knee ligaments. Instead of stresses being absorbed by muscle, they are transferred to ligaments.

Playing style

Females often play in an upright position which may cause considerable stress to the knee. A body position born from the athletic posture, bent at the knees and hips, better absorbs the shock of feet pounding and maneuvering on turf.

Lack of neuromuscular control

Current evidence suggests that the primary reason girls are at risk is that girls have less neuromuscular control of knee motion during athletic play. There are specific ways that girls use their muscles that lead to dynamic knee valgus (knees bending inward or knock-kneed). When knees are out of alignment in this fashion there's a high risk of ACL tearing.

1. **Girls use quadriceps muscles much more than hamstrings** and as a result strain the ACL. Strain is reduced when there is a co-contraction of the hamstrings (when both quads and hamstrings work together).

2. **Girls tend to have one leg stronger than the other** that results in uneven weight distribution between the feet upon landing. This causes the body's center of mass to move away from its base of support — a position associated with increased risk of ACL injury.

3. **Girls tend to have less core strength and stability.** Having less control of their center of mass, they cannot prevent it from shifting away from the base of support.

4. **Girls tend to use bones and ligaments to stop motion**, rather than contracting muscles to control joint position and absorb landing forces.

The good news is neuromuscular risk factors may be changed for the better through training.

Importance of training

It has been asserted by some that males get a much earlier start in athletics than females. Boys are trained at younger ages in activities that have increased their strength, agility, coordination and proprioception (the body's ability to sense the movement and position of muscles without visual guides — essential for any activity requiring hand-eye coordination).

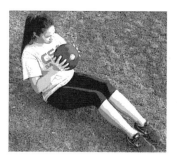

Along with skills training, boys have been encouraged to pursue strength and conditioning programs that will enhance performance and help prevent injury. Girls are not likewise encouraged until much later on, if at all. Even in today's new world there is a mindset (in some places) that strength and conditioning programs are not for girls.

It can be argued that boys get better coaching and training from the get go. Without strong leaders and direction, females miss out on appropriate training that may very well prevent injury and build better athletes.

Preventing ACL injuries in female athletes

There is evidence that neuromuscular training (NMT) programs can reduce lower-extremity injuries. Neuromuscular pertains to the interplay between nerves and muscles. Such training strengthens hamstring, quadriceps and core (trunk) muscles, develops balance, and teaches girls how to identify and steer clear of dynamic knee valgus (knees buckling inward during athletic movement).

For the greater part, training consists of a step-by-step strengthening of the legs and core, plyometrics (jumping exercises) and technique development through hands-on coaching. It is also important that programs improve flexibility, balance and agility. Training is covered more fully in the next chapters.

Strengthening

Exercises such as squats and lunges target the thigh and gluteal muscles and hip external rotators — muscle groups that work to counteract hip and leg movements that cause dynamic knee valgus.

Exercises such as planks and prone lifts work on core strength as well as hamstrings and gluteal muscles.

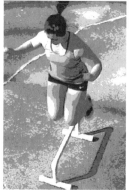

Plyometrics
These are repeated jumping exercises in which leg muscles rapidly contract from a stretched position with maximum force thus increasing muscle power.

Exercises include two-legged takeoffs and landings or squat jumps. Athletes may then graduate to one-legged takeoffs and landings — hopping or bounding, in place from one leg to the other.

Technique development
There needs to be a coach involved who is specifically trained in recognizing dynamic knee valgus. The instructor teaches athletes to know exactly what that is and how to avoid it. Proper form is coached and developed through ever greater exercise challenges.

Athletes are constantly encouraged to keep knees over feet (not knocked-kneed) and to land softly — that is, with legs flexed to absorb the shock of landing from jumps.

Timing, frequency and duration

Studies show that the best time to begin NMT programs is during early adolescence. A minimum of six to eight weeks of training is needed before neuromuscular changes are seen and athletic performance improves — a minimum of twice per week for six weeks.

Integrating NMT programs into daily physical education classes would extend the benefits of such training to girls involved in recreational physical activities as well as competitive sports.

Resources for NMT programs

Sportsmetrics: www.sportsmetrics.org

PEP (Prevent injury, Enhance Performance): www.smsmf.org/smsf-programs/pep-program

KIPP (Knee Injury Prevention Program) for Coaches: http://kipp.instituteforsportsmedicine.org

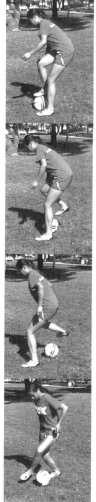

Moving like a boy

"Silvers directed my attention to one more player, a girl who seemed light on her feet, quick and springy. When she changed directions, she stayed in what generations of gym teachers have called 'the athletic position' — knees bent, butt low to the ground. Even when walking casually during stoppages in play, she seemed more lithe than the other girls. "She moves more like a boy," Silvers said. "Believe me, that's a good thing."

From an article in the *New York Times Magazine*, "The Uneven Playing Field" by Michael Sokolove published May 11, 2008. Holly Silvers, a physical therapist and the director of research at the Santa Monica Orthopaedic and Sports Medicine Research Foundation, is quoted. Silvers and Sokolove were watching an elite girls soccer match, and Silvers was reviewing the playing style of various players.

Before her injuries, Joy could kick it around some.

Sources for *ACL overview, Girls & ACLs* and *Quick reference*

American Orthopaedic Society for Sports Medicine. *Anterior Cruciate Ligament (ACL) Injuries,* http://orthoinfo.aaos.org/topic.cfm?topic=a00549 (March 2014).

American Orthopaedic Society for Sports Medicine. *Knee Arthroscopy,* http://orthoinfo.aaos.org/topic.cfm?topic=a00299 (March 2010).

Boatright, Dr. *Knee Injuries in Female Athletes,* http://www.drrickboatright.com/blog/2012/11/knee-injuries-in-female-athletes/ (November 2012).

Chiaia, Theresa PT and de Mille, Polly RN, MA, RCEP, CSCS. *ACL Injury Prevention Tips and Exercises: Stay Off the Sidelines!* http://www.hss.edu/conditions_acl-injury-prevention-stay-off-sidelines.asp#.VPTb5EZ3z8U (March 2009).

Dharamsi, Aisha MD and LaBella, Cynthia MD. *Prevention of ACL Injuries in Adolescent Female Athletes,* http://contemporarypediatrics.modernmedicine.com/contemporary-pediatrics/content/tags/acl-injury/prevention-acl-injuries-adolescent-female-athletes?page=full (July 2013).

Hofmann, Margaret. *Why Women Should Train Differently From Men,* http://www.femaleathletesfirst.com/ArticlesFAQs/TheFemaleAthlete/TabId/124/ArtMID/457/ArticleID/23/Why-Women-Should-Train-Differently-From-Men.aspx (September 2012).

Kim, Jennifer and Smith, Joe. *Anterior Cruciate Ligament Injury (ACL),* http://orthosurg.ucsf.edu/patient-care/divisions/sports-medicine/conditions/knee/anterior-cruciate-ligament-injury-acl/#.VGKp3UZ3y6U (January 2009).

Mary Ann Porucznik. *Athletes Risk Second ACL Injury After ACL Reconstruction,* http://www.aaos.org/news/aaosnow/aug13/clinical1.asp (August 2013).

MedicineNet. *Definition of Neuromuscular,* http://www.medicinenet.com/script/main/art.asp?articlekey=34038 (June 2012).

Shultz, S. J. *Sex differences in knee joint laxity change across the female menstrual cycle,* http://www.ncbi.nlm.nih.gov/pmc/articles/PMC1890029/ (December 2005).

Skinner, H.B. MD, PhD. *Exercise-related knee joint laxity,* http://ajs.sagepub.com/content/14/1/30.abstract

Sokolove, Michael. "The Uneven Playing Field," *New York Times Magazine* (May, 2008).

Souryal, Tarek O. M.D. *ACL Injury, ACL Tear, ACL Surgery,* http://www.txsportsmed.com/acl.php

Trayl Body Work. *Knee pain Tibial external rotation syndrome,* http://traylbodywork.com/video/knee-pain-tibial-external-rotation-syndrome/ (August 2012).

Virginia Commonwealth University. *Unit VI – The Hip,* http://www.courses.vcu.edu/DANC291-003/unit_6.htm

Wilkerson, Rick DO. Arthroscopy, http://orthoinfo.aaos.org/topic.cfm?topic=a00109 (May 2010).

Wong, Eric. *Knee Stability and Punching Power (Part 1),* http://ericwongmma.com/knee-stability-and-punching-power-part-1

6. *How to rehab*
What our PT has to say

Patience, compliance, consistency
The most important things a patient should understand about their rehab process can be broken down into three words: patience, compliance and consistency.

Patience

A patient has to understand that the healing process is long, especially after surgery. With an ACL surgery, the visible remnants of a standard procedure are four to five little scars. What she does not see is the amount of tissue cut and bone drilled underneath. These deep wounds take several weeks to fully heal. The body wants to heal — it's designed to — but it takes time, patience and the acceptance that pain will be a regular ordeal for several weeks.

Compliance

Because the healing process is slow and gradual, compliance to the correct exercises at the correct stages of healing are essential. In the first stages of rehab, the muscles in the knee are very weak due to immobility and the physical traumas of surgery. Because of the lack of muscular support, the knee is very unstable, and the risk or reinjury to the newly repaired ACL is high. It is important to stay compliant with the given exercises at the recommended frequency in order to not overstress the muscles or ligaments, and to maximize the amount of strengthening of the muscles in preparation for more advanced exercises in the future. This applies to the later stages in rehab as well. Compliance while performing the higher level exercises is crucial to maximize the rehab potential.

Consistency
Compliance and consistency tend to go hand in hand and the most successful rehab patients are the ones that combine the two. A patient can be compliant with doing the exercises, but may not be doing them as frequently as they should; or they may be consistently performing them incorrectly. It is my experience that the most successful patients are the ones that put in a lot of effort to perform their recommended exercises at home at the recommended frequency, not just during their one or two physical therapy visits each week.

A good patient consistently asks questions and gives feedback to the therapist about how the knee feels with certain activities. Patients who consistently perform the exercises correctly and make the effort to adjust their form after feedback from the therapist are typically the ones who have the most success.

How to cope

I find education and positive reinforcement to be the best way for me to help patients mentally with their rehabilitation.

Education is key in giving patients peace of mind. Patients need to be informed about every aspect of their condition, including what is injured, how to prevent reinjury, how long it may possibly take to heal and what it will take to optimize healing. Often just understanding the process of rehab gives patients some peace of mind. The more informed a patient is about why things hurt, the less anxiety the patients will have about it hurting. This allows the focus to be shifted toward their rehab.

Secondly, I tend to go with a positive approach when progressing patients through their rehab program. I make it known to the patient when range of motion increases and when performance and quality of exercise improves. It's a cause for celebration when patients report being able to do daily tasks that they were not able to do before.

I enjoy being the cheerleader, and patients tend to respond well to someone who is rooting for them to get better. When a patient discovers that their range of motion has increased from a week ago or that they are now able to lift a five-pound weight when they could only lift three pounds just three days ago, she is able to see physical improvement. This encourages the patients to continue their hard work and builds trust in the program and in me.

Dr. Justin Balleza, DPT

The next two chapters outline the rehab process as prescribed by Dr. Balleza after Joy's second ACL injury.

7. *Joy's rehab*
First six months

<u>Stage 1:</u> *Swelling management and basic strengthening*

Swelling Management: P-R-I-C-E
P — Protect by wearing a knee brace (except for sleeping)
R — Rest
I — Ice two to three times each day, 10-15 minutes at a time
C — Compression
E — Elevate

Passive ROM (Range of Motion)
● In a long sitting position, center a small towel under the foot of the affected leg. Grasp the ends of the towel on either side of the foot and leg. Gently pull the foot closer to the buttocks and bend the knee.

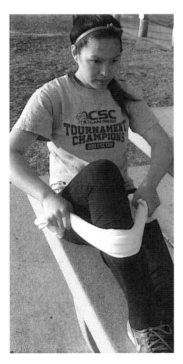

● Find a mildly uncomfortable end range and hold for 3-5 seconds.

● Try to bend the knee farther with every repetition, but not exceeding a mildly uncomfortable feeling. The exercise should not be very painful.

Low level strengthening exercises performed with protective knee brace
● *Quad sets* — Tense the quads making sure the knee cap moves up and holds 3-5 seconds each time to "wake up" the quadriceps in preparation for more advanced exercises.

● Straight leg raises (three ways) — These exercises help strengthen the anterior and lateral aspects of the knee in preparation for more weight bearing activities during Stage 2.

1. *Supine (lying on back) position:* With the leg completely extended, lift the leg 12-20 inches off the floor. Then lower it in a slow, controlled manner.

2. *Side-lying abduction (moving leg outwardly, away from center):* The affected leg should be facing up toward the ceiling. Lift the leg 12-20 inches off the floor, then lower slowly in a controlled manner.

3. *Side-lying adduction (moving leg inwardly):* The injured leg should be touching the surface of the floor/table. Lift the affected leg 6-10 inches off the floor, then lower in the prescribed manner.

Precautions
Avoid Long Arc Quad (LAQ) exercises (lifting the leg through a 90-degree arch in a supine position). Due to a lack of quad strength and healing, this exercise may reinjure the ACL.

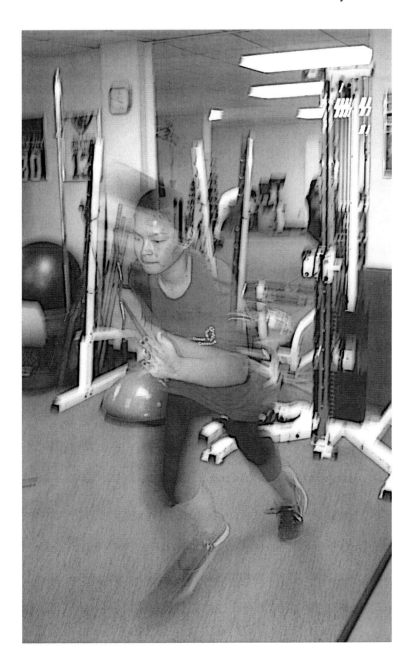

Stage 2: Weight bearing activities and intermediate strengthening

Stationary bike, 5-10 minutes
● Use little to no resistance to warm up the joint, increase circulation in the area, activate quads and hamstrings and help reduce swelling.

Short Arc Quads (SAQ)
Here the leg lifts through an arch less than a 90-degree arch in a supine position.
● Place a 6-10 inch bolster underneath your knee. Activate the quadriceps to straighten the knee and slowly lower the leg. Repeat.

Mini squats progressing to conventional squats
● Support yourself with hands on a table. Put equal pressure into both legs and bend your knees about 20-30 degrees. Slowly straighten back to a normal standing position. Keep your quads and glutes tense throughout the entire exercise. Feet should be in a neutral, front-facing position and shoulder-width apart.

● Progress to a 90-degree bend when you can tolerate the sharper angle.

One-foot leg press
● Exercise with low resistance and in a supine/gravity-eliminated position.

● Place the foot of the affected leg on the platform and bend the knee slowly in a controlled manner with active effort to reduce knee wobble. The knee should be bent to about 90 degrees, then straightened at a slow and comfortable pace.

Straight leg raise three ways
Supine, side abduction and side adduction
● Continue with a steady progression of increased ankle weight to develop strength and muscle activation.

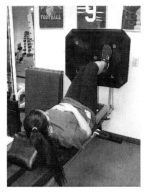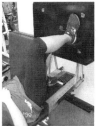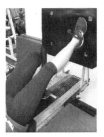

One-foot leg presses

Straight leg raises:
three ways with weights

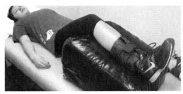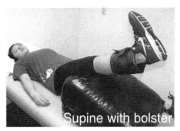

Supine with bolster

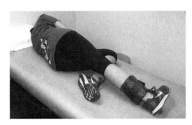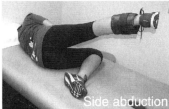

Side abduction

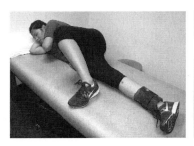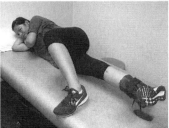

Stage 3: Dynamic strengthening and stabilization

Resisted walks
● Using a weighted pulley machine, attach the waist strap.
● Starting with light weight and a slow gait, walk against the resistance of the pulley to the end of the cable. Walk backward slowly and return to the starting point.
● Progress with increased weight and a faster pace.
● *Advanced:* with heavy weight, perform alternating lunges to the end range of the cable.

Balance board
● This wooden board rocks from side to side like a see-saw and trains you to begin putting equal pressure into both legs with closed-chain activities.
● Stand with each foot an equal distance from center on top of the platform.
● Rock the board side to side and allow each end to touch the floor softly and slowly. This exercise requires constant readjustment of both quadriceps muscles to make the side-to-side motion smooth and the touchdowns soft.

Lunges over Dyna Discs
● Using the affected leg, step on top of a Dyna Disc (an unsteady, air-inflated plate) and perform a lunge, keeping the knee and ankle as steady as possible over the wobbly surface.
● This allows you to actively stabilize the ankle and knee during a functional movement that requires the recruitment of hip, knee and ankle musculature.

Bosu Ball squats
● Turn the Bosu Ball upside down.
● Stand and balance on top of the flat surface of the Bosu using hand supports to ensure safety.
● Once you feel steady, start the squats. Depth will vary on how well you perform the task.
● Squatting on top of the Bosu requires that you put equal pressure to both knees in order to keep the Bosu in a neutral position.

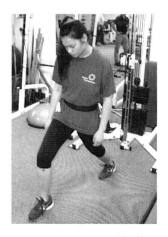

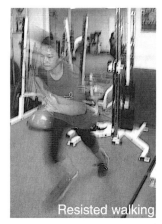

Resisted walking

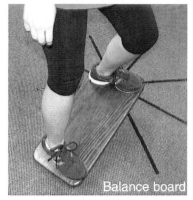

Balance board

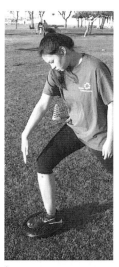

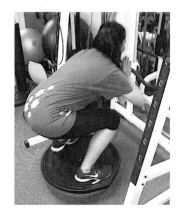

Lunges over a Dyna Disc (above) and squats with a Bosu Ball (left) require the use of of a variety of muscles to maintain stability.

Stage 4: *Plyometrics, cutting and return to sport*
At this stage, the patient has achieved good quadriceps strength, knee pain is very minimal and the repaired ACL has had about 4-6 months of healing since surgery.

Running program
● At this point you should be running regularly with a gradual progression in pace and distance.

Leg press one-legged hops
● Using low resistance, the patient is eased into plyometrics using the horizontal leg press with low weight. This allows the patient to adapt to heavier impact at a lower intensity than would be the case with vertical jumping without gear.

● Progress by increasing weight.

Box jumps
● Increase the height of the box as you improve. Land lightly on the forefoot rather than flat footed to mitigate the shock from the foot to the knees

Cone exercises: Lateral shuffles
● Here you perform heel-clicks or defensive slides side to side between spaced cones. Maintain an athletic stance at all times!

● This exercise is meant to get you used to cutting again and to build confidence in the healing knee. These shuffles allow the body to adapt to lateral motion and deceleration of lateral movement as weight is shifted to change direction.

Floor ladder exercises
● *High knees*: Very similar to the football drill where players step through and over tires. Here we are using a floor ladder with instructions to keep knees high and steps light and quick.

● This exercise is performed laterally and forward.

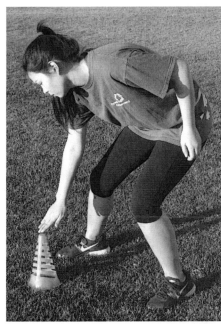

Lateral shuffles exercise the demands of weight shifting and changing of direction — the essence of cutting.

Ladder exercises improve agility — stepping quickly, lightly and accurately. Keep those knees high!

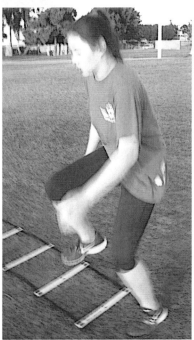

Notes from our PT

Various manual techniques such as patellar mobilization (moving the kneecap), effleurage (massage) to decrease swelling, passive and prolonged stretching and constant instruction on form with all exercises are key to a successful rehabilitation. Modalities such as Neuromuscular Electrical Stimulation (NMES), ice and sports wraps are also regularly used in the rehabilitation process (opposite page).

A trained set of eyes that continuously catches compensations, muscular imbalances, proper foot, knee, hip and low back positioning with each exercise helps the patient restore full function to the knee.

Muscle strength is not the only aspect that must be prioritized during this rehabilitation. Making sure the leg musculature does not develop imbalances (tight hamstrings or calves, weak gluteal muscles, tight adductors or hip external rotators) is important to minimize compensations that could lead to injury or reinjury.

A neurological aspect must also be considered. How quickly does the body adapt to external forces (perturbations, uneven surfaces, hard landings or slippery surfaces)? Has the body been trained to react to such external factors?

And lastly, the psychological aspect of the patient must be addressed. Is the patient confident that the knee will not get reinjured? Is the patient willing to return to the activity she enjoys doing? The patient should feel comfortable performing the advanced exercises in Stage 4. Proper encouragement, instruction and a gradual progression are key to improving the mindset of the athlete.

Stage 4 exercises along with the dynamic balance exercises in Stage 3 are great exercises in helping to prevent ACL injuries. Muscle strength and the ability to adapt to unsteady external forces may help prevent injury.

Dr. Justin Balleza, DPT

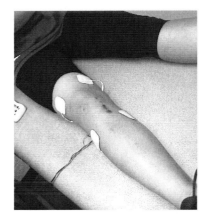

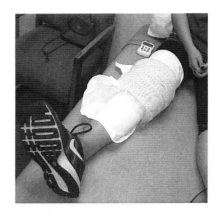

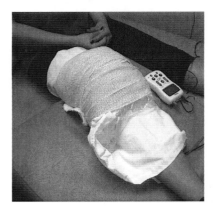

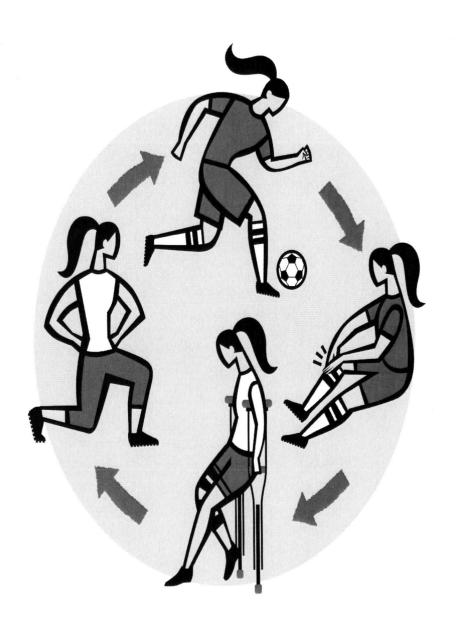

8. *Advanced*
Training beyond rehab

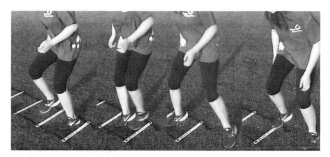

Agility ladder drills

Two-feet-in pattern moving forward
● When performing this exercise, each foot should land in the same box before moving on to the next box.

● Exercises should be performed quickly with a symmetrical step time and landing.

● Each foot should land forefoot first to reduce shock through the joints.

● When this exercise is performed correctly, you should appear to be performing swift high knees moving forward. The ladder is only meant to give guidance where to land each foot.

Two-feet-in pattern moving laterally
● The same pattern is performed as the forward pattern, but the patient should be moving laterally through the boxes.

● This should be performed moving laterally to the right as well as the left to prevent any imbalances or compensations.

These ladder drills can be progressed with more complicated patterns which can be found in various source material (internet/instruction manual of agility ladder).

Line drills

Suicides
● Suicides are a common drill in which the athlete sprints up and down a field or court.

● Using a marked soccer field, basketball court, parking lot or the like, use the marked lines to determine when to decelerate, change direction and sprint back to the starting line.

● Sprint back from the first marked line, return to the starting line and sprint to a line marked further than the first.

● Deceleration is the key part of this exercise. Be sure to practice changing directions using both the right and the left with a particular bias using the repaired ACL side more in order to acclimate to cutting on that affected side

● Each change of direction should be performed with control and progressed with a more explosive takeoff as tolerated.

Heel clicks
● The same forward and back pattern as the suicide drill can be used with this exercise, increasing the distance to return to the starting line with every round.

● The difference is that we are focusing on lateral motion, a common movement in many field sports (defensive slides, cutting, etc).

● You should be in a defensive stance (hips and knees slightly bent, wide stance).

● Take off laterally in a galloping motion, making sure to "click" the heels with every cycle.

● Again, this exercise should be performed in symmetry, making sure lateral motion is performed going left and right.

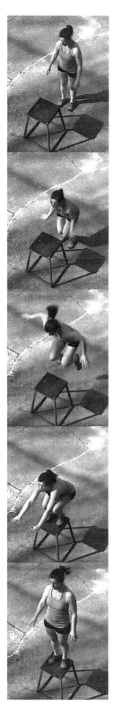

Plyometric exercises

Box jumps

● This exercise works on explosiveness.

● This should be started with a short box (no higher than two feet).

● The athlete jumps with a symmetrical takeoff and lands lightly on the forefoot onto the box. The repetition is finished with the athlete hopping back down from the box, back to the starting position (also landing softly).

● This can be progressed with increased box height as well as increasing the swiftness of each repetition.

Switch kicks

● This can be performed using a box, bench or nothing at all.

● The athlete alternates a small jump kick quickly.

● Use a bench/box to tap the kicking foot before the kicking foot lands — the planted foot should already be hopping into the kick.

● This can be performed using a timer or a set amount of repetitions, but should be done quickly and symmetrically.

High knee skips
● This exercise can be performed in an open field or court.

● Skips are similar to that of a basketball layup in which the athlete skips down the field at a determined distance, alternating each jumping foot with every repetition. The non-jumping foot should be performing a high knee, making sure the knee is at least above the waistline before coming back down.

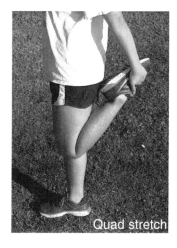

Quad stretch

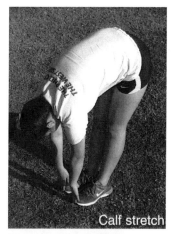

Calf stretch

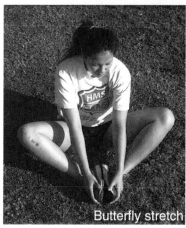

Butterfly stretch

Stretches

Quad stretch
● A common stretch and effective for stretching the quadriceps.

● Standing on one foot, bring the stretching foot back toward the butt and grab the foot with the hand of the same side.

● Use the hand to pull the foot in an upward/forward direction until the stretch is felt in the front thigh.

● Stretches should be held for a minimum of 20-30 seconds.

● If balance is an issue, use the non-stretching hand for support from a wall or rail.

Hamstring stretch
● There are many ways to stretch the hamstrings including reaching down to touch the toes without bending the knees, reaching forward in a long-sitting position to touch the toes, or having someone lift a straight leg in a lying position. All are effective stretches for the hamstrings.

● Stretch each hamstring for a minimum of 20-30 seconds.

Butterfly stretch
● In a sitting position, have the soles of each feet touch each other.

● Use both hands to pull the feet toward the groin until a mild stretch is felt.

● Increase the stretch by using both elbows to push down into the knees in the butterfly position (spreading the wings).

● The stretch should be felt in the groin/inner thigh.

● Hold 20-30 seconds.

Torn

Calf stretch

● Leaning against a wall using both hands, position into a split stance and straighten out the back leg.

● Lean forward until the stretch is felt in the upper calf (gastrocnemius muscle). Make sure to keep the heel of the back leg down.

● After 20-30 seconds, slightly bend the knee of the back leg. A stretch should be felt in the lower part of the calf (soleus muscle).

● Hold for another 20-30 seconds, then switch stance and repeat.

9. *Training*
for girl athletes

Except for a select few, girls do not get real athletic conditioning before they hit the playing field. Most girls are not lucky enough to enjoy enlightened programs and coaches; or talented enough for the elite programs to recruit; or knowledgeable enough to find the training on their own.

In most cases it goes like this: families read the flyers, have their girls show up on a given date and try out — *Let's see whatcha got!* Hopefully the coach calls up *because you made the team!* and tells you when and where to start practice.

Practice is all about skill drills, some playing and, of course, getting in shape. Coach wants to determine whose best right away in order to build the best team she can in the window of time allotted. She also wants to develop more skilled players in general and make sure players can play strong throughout the game.

It's the latter that may not be addressed as urgently and *thoroughly* as the rest.

> There are girls out there ready to play, but there are lots of girls who are not.

Conditioning is often considered a by-product of simply showing up at each practice and working hard. However, the kind of conditioning this book advocates takes the kind of time, thought and effort *always* given to talent search and development.

There are girls out there ready to play, but there are lots of girls who are not. They do not know how to move athletically. They do not have the wherewithal to move with strength, effectiveness and assurance. They lack flexibility, sufficiently strong legs and core, balance and agility. And as odd as it may sound, many girls don't know how to jump and land safely.

This does not mean they cannot play — a certain lack of physical fitness and grace can be overcome by desire, for example. But it does mean they have physical shortcomings that mitigate performance and *allow for injury.*

Regimen

Starting on page 116 are training exercises. They are divided into five categories:

1. Strength core
2. Strength legs
3. Explosiveness (plyometrics)
4. Agility
5. Balance
6. Flexibility

Work all six categories of training two to three times a week. Everybody is different so reps and sets will differ from athlete to athlete. But work hard to improve. If you do this stuff you will be a better athlete and better equipped to prevent injury.

Strength core
At least twice a week. Pick any two that work different muscles. Mix them up from week to week. Eight to ten reps, three sets. Hold the plank exercises for at least 30 seconds times three. Remember if the exercise works one leg or side, you gotta work the other!

Strength legs
Same as core.

Plyometrics
At least twice a week. Pick one and work it. Several jumps in sets of three.

Agility
Pick one. At least twice a week. Mix it up. Several minutes each.

Balance
Spend some time with one at least twice a week.

Flexibility
Stretch before and after workouts. Hold for 20-30 seconds.

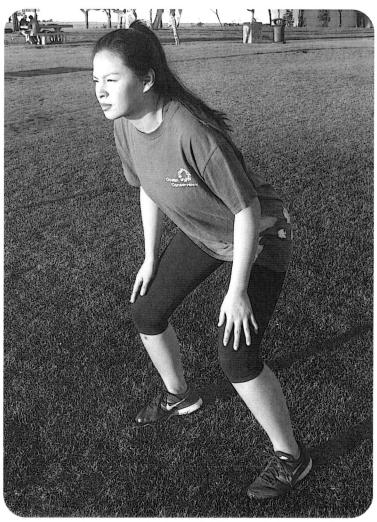

The first position in athletic movement.

Athletic stance

It begins and ends — all proper athletic movement — with the athletic stance. It's astonishing that something so vital to sport — ALL sports — is overlooked in so many programs for girls. But it is. And it is our contention that committing the ready position to muscle memory — making it automatic — will pave the way to safer and more effective performance.

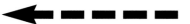

Feet point straight ahead. Weight on balls of feet. Bend knees so they are out over your toes. Arch back, bend at the waist and stick out your butt so that the angle of your back matches the angle of your shins. Chest out, shoulders pinched. Shoulders over knees over feet. Head up, eyes forward.

From an athletic stance you are ready to move in any direction. Ready to *spring* in any direction with force. Energy is effectively transferred from nerves to muscle tissue — not through joints and ligaments. If you learn to begin and end every move you make with the ready position, you are halfway there.

Exercises

The rest of the way includes an ongoing plan of action that builds core and leg strength, explosiveness, agility, balance and flexibility. Sounds like a lot and it does take a fair amount of time and effort that may or may not be an expected part of a typical high school soccer or lacrosse program.

It's important to understand that such a program has it's own requirements and does not overlap with the drills, scrimmages and goings on of most practices. It's its own thing and must be respected as much as anything else put on a young athlete's plate. The tendency has been to plug in the conditioning when convenient, always making way for skill development and playing time.

1. Strength exercises: core

When we are talking about developing core strength, we are referring to the conditioning of abdominal and back muscles and those muscles around the pelvis. The most important thing a strong core will do is enable an athlete to keep her weight centered and balanced over legs and feet. Athletic movement will be hindered, sloppy and unsafe if girls cannot change direction without losing their center.

Pick up and reach

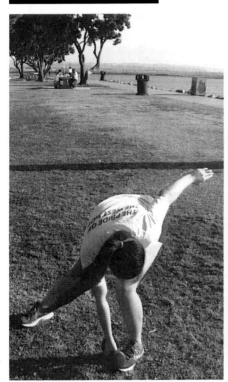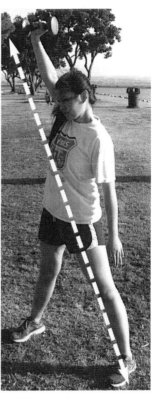

Joy bends her left knee and extends the weight over her left
foot. She then brings the weight across herself and reaches it
above her right shoulder. Joy uses a light dumbbell, about five
pounds.

Push up plank with kicks

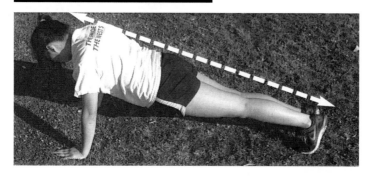

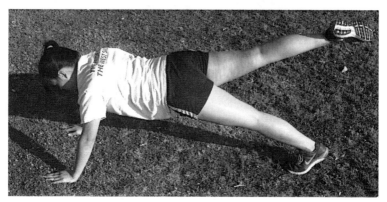

Joy begins with a plank supported by straight arms — like a pushup. Back, hips and legs form a straight line. While holding the plank, she lifts her leg up, out and up and over.

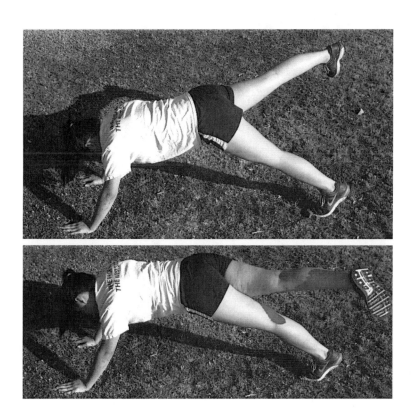

Kettlebell squat to overhead swings

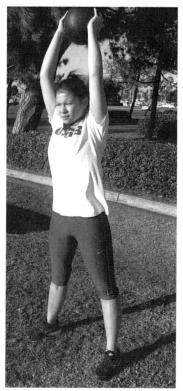 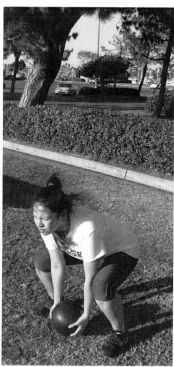

Joy does a squat and brings the weight between her knees. Then she sweeps the ball up and directly over her head. The ball in these images is a ten-pound slam ball.

Four-way X-chop

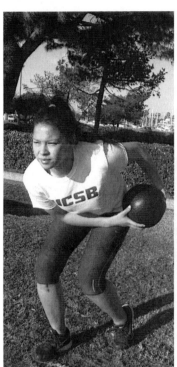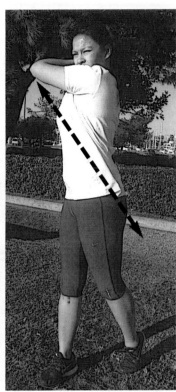

With one foot leading the other, Joy bends at the knees and waist and brings the ball to her left hip. She then rotates and swings the ball up and over her right shoulder. You make an **X** when you work both sides.

Weighted Russian twist

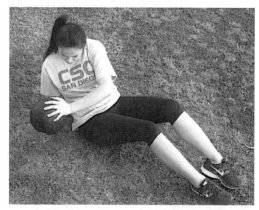

From a sitting position, Joy bends her knees and leans slightly back. Here she is holding a weighted ball, but the exercise can be done without weight. While holding the position (with back straight!) she rotates her trunk to each side.

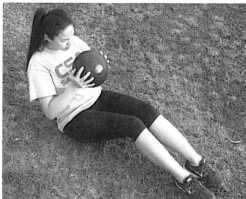

Lift heels to increase difficulty.

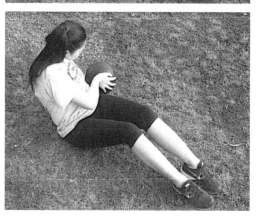

Ball slams

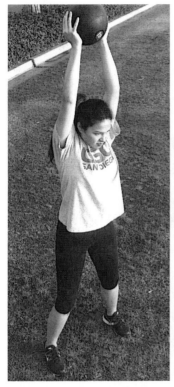
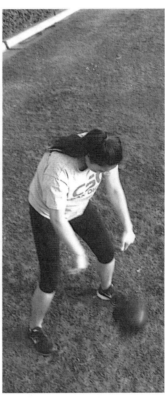

Joy sweeps the ten-pound slam ball directly overhead and slams it into the turf. Perhaps the most cathartic of all exercises!

Pushups

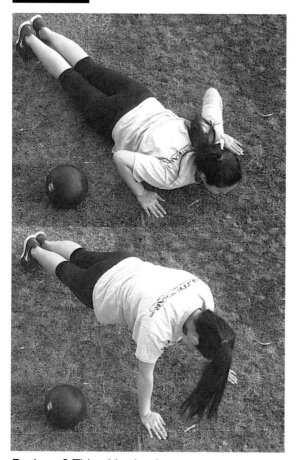

Pushups? This old school
exercise does more than work
the arms. From the straight-
back position, Joy lowers herself to her chest. For
beginners, start the plank
from the knees.

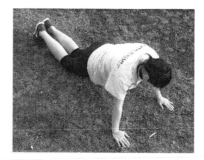

Planks

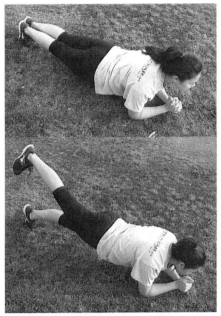

Holding the body in a straight line is key. In the top two images Joy is holding a plank on her elbows and raising a leg.

The bottom images show her maintaining a rigid position from her side. Legs are raised straight from the hips.

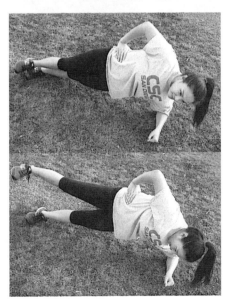

Hamstring curls

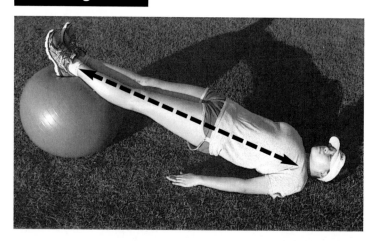

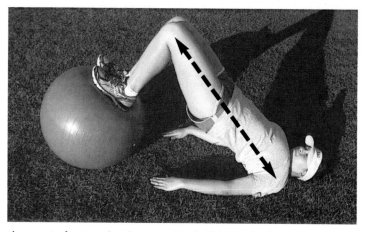

Joy rests feet and calves on the ball in a plank position and pulls the ball toward her butt maintaining a straight line from knees to chin.

2. Strength exercises: legs

Here squats, lunges and variations thereof predominate. The goal is to punch up quadriceps and hamstrings — the most important muscles for knee support.

Squats

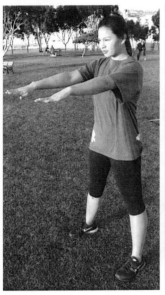 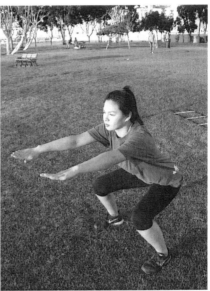

Joy lowers herself with back straight, knees over or behind toes, hips below parallel and weight on heels.

Half or quarter squats for those early in rehab.

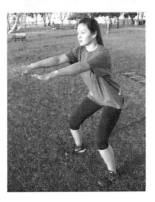

Weighted squats

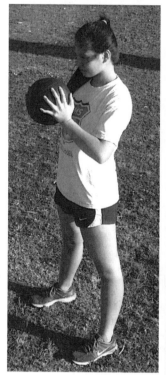 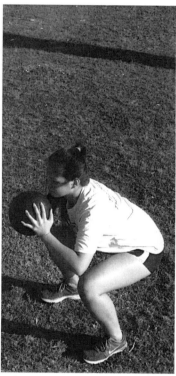

Squatting with the medicine ball.

Lunges

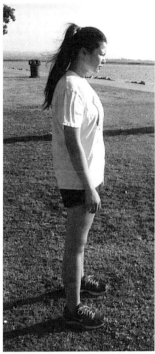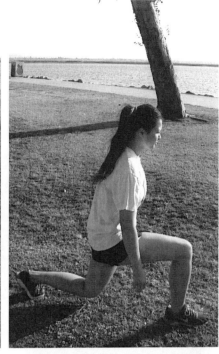

Joy makes a stride and lowers herself so that her knee brushes the turf or deck. Back is straight. Add the weight for more fun.

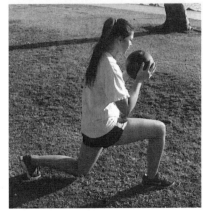

Single leg step ups

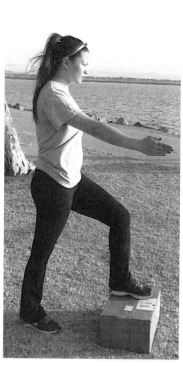 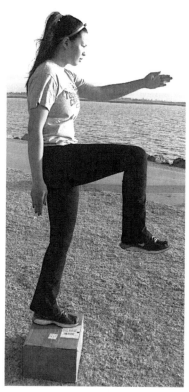

Step on a box or curb with one leg. Thrust the opposite knee up in line with hip and shoulder. Arms swing opposite to stepping legs. Bring the thrusting leg down to touch the turf or deck and immediately begin another thrust. Increase the height of the box as you progress.

This exercise builds strength and balance.

Weighted step ups

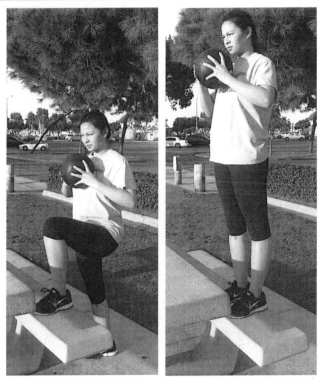

As shown. Maintain an upright posture throughout.

Single leg retro squats

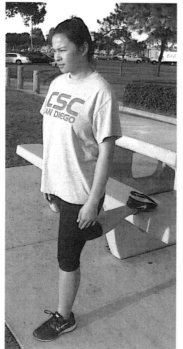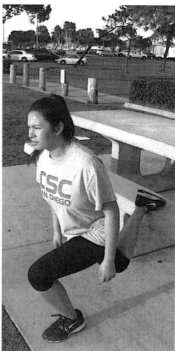

Like lunges, but also works stabilizing muscles.

3. Exercises for explosiveness

Learning how to jump is not as ridiculous as it may seem. There is a technique to doing it effectively. And drilling the following exercises will develop a powerful coordination between quadriceps and hamstring muscles essential for athletic thrust.

Squat jumps

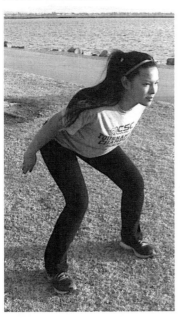
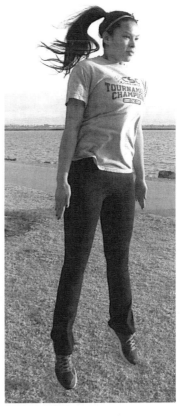

From a squat, jump straight up. Strive to thrust equally off both legs and to land softly on the balls of your feet with knees flexed. Your take off and landing positions should look alike.

Low hurdle hops

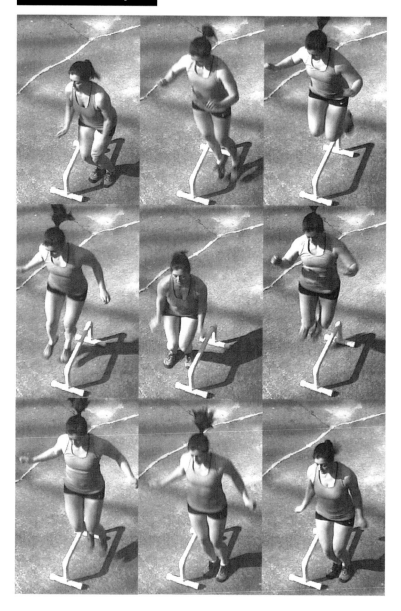

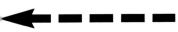

Here we use a hurdle, but any 12-inch barrier will do. Standing next to the hurdle, Kylie hops to the other side always using a two-footed hop with the feet close together (not merely stepping over the hurdle).

Note the symmetry of her technique. Kylie is aligned from shoulders to hips to knees to ankles. Knees are bent to absorb shock and then thrust.

Land like a feather

"Learn how to move with good alignment so you protect your knees. Develop body awareness, strength and balance to support your knees and ankles. Always jump, land, stop and move with your knees directly over your feet. Do NOT let your knees collapse inward.

"Say to yourself:
Chest high and over knees
Bend from the hips and knees
Knees over toes
Toes straight forward
Land like a feather"

Directly quoted from an article by Theresa Chiala and Polly de Mille, *ACL Injury Prevention Tips and Exercises: Stay Off the Sidelines!*

http://www.hss.edu/conditions_acl-injury-prevention-stay-off-sidelines.asp#.VPTb5EZ3z8U (March 2009)

Box jumps

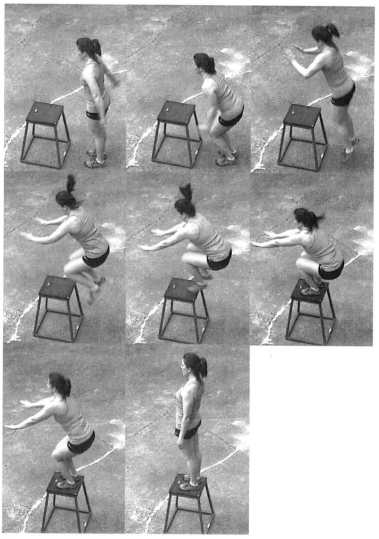

This box is high for beginners. Start lower
to perfect technique. Again, note the symmetry and alignment. Kylie is in balance
and in control. No flailing limbs!

4. Agility exercises

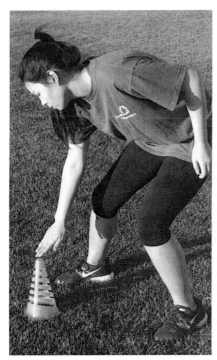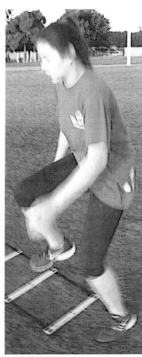

Cone touches

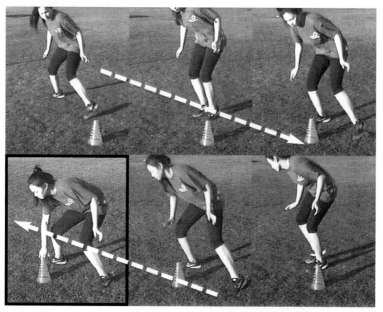

This exercise works lateral motion, deceleration and cutting thrust. The idea is to gain ever greater control and confidence with explosive changes in direction.

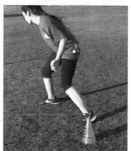

Ladder steps

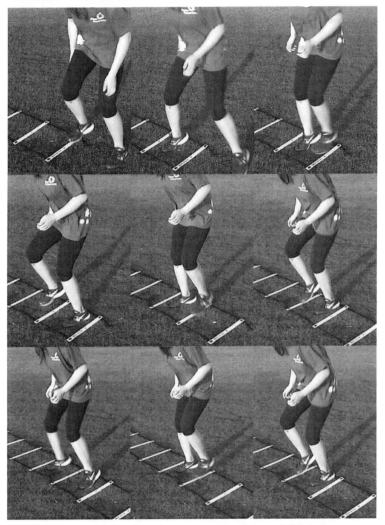

Ladder steps require that Joy execute quick and light steps accurately.

5. Balancing exercises

Leg reaches

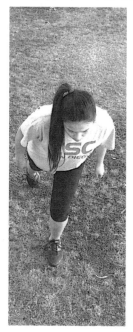
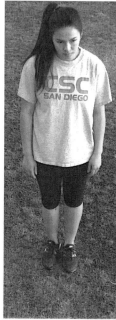
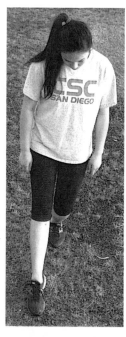

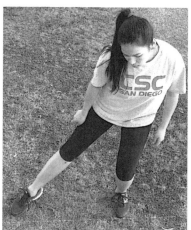
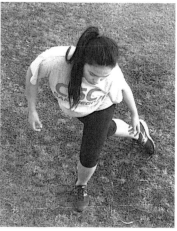

Balancing on one leg, Joy reaches forward, back, right and left.

Balancing board

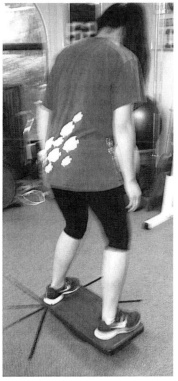

Joy's goal is to maintain balance and control while slowly touching each end of the board to the deck.

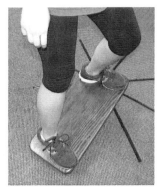

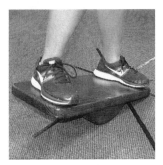

Bosu Ball squats

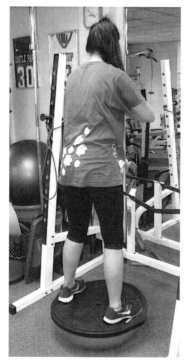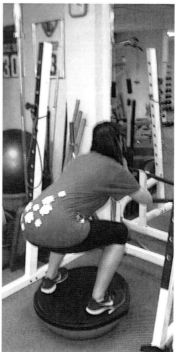

Successful squats on the Bosu Ball will require that Joy use both legs equally to maintain balance.

Dead lift

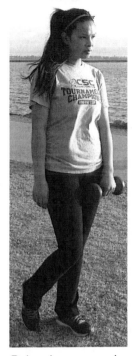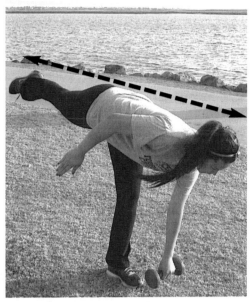

Balancing on one leg, Joy slowly reaches with a light dumbbell and swings her opposite leg up and back. The lifted leg is straight throughout. Leg and back make a straight line at the apex.

6. Stretches for flexibility

Quad

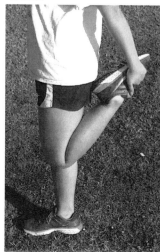

Hamstring

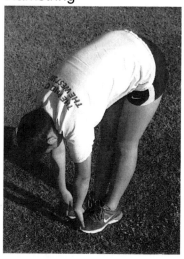

Butterfly

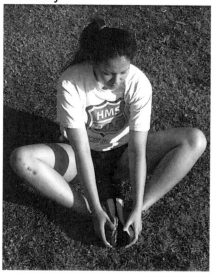

Sources for *Training*

Chiaia, Theresa PT and de Mille, Polly RN, MA, RCEP, CSCS. *ACL Injury Prevention Tips and Exercises: Stay Off the Sidelines!* http://www.hss.edu/conditions_acl-injury-prevention-stay-off-sidelines.asp#.VPTb5EZ3z8U (March 2009).

Hatmaker, Kylie and Hatmaker, Mark. *She's Tough.* San Diego, CA: Tracks Publishing, 2014.

Mayo Clinic. *Core exercises build abs and other core muscles,* http://www.mayoclinic.org/healthy-living/fitness/multimedia/core-strength/sls-20076575

National Academy of Sports Medicine. *What are good cues to teach the common athletic position?* http://www.sharecare.com/health/football/what-good-teach-athletic-position

Safe Kids Worldwide. *Game Changers: 7 Exercises to Prevent ACL Injuries,* http://www.safekids.org/acltraining

Shaw, Jene. *Ditch Your Crunches,* http://triathlon.competitor.com/2013/04/training/ditch-your-crunches_52216 (April 2015)

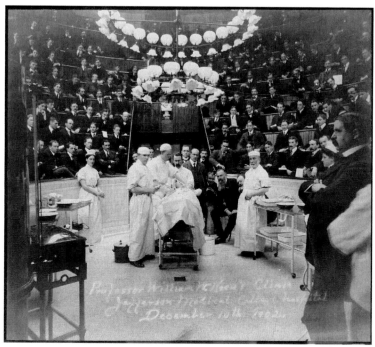

Your knee surgery will be much less intrusive and a great deal less complicated than in years past. Library of Congress.

10. FAQs
A quick reference

What is an ACL?

ACL stands for anterior cruciate ligament. It is the most important ligament in the knee. It connects the thigh bone to the shine bone. When it tears, the leg loses its stability. It does not heal. When this ligament tears, it must be replaced if you want to play again.

The more boyish the build (slim hips aligned over knees and feet, strong core and legs) — the better ...

What causes it to tear or break?

Most ACL injuries occur during athletic play. The foot is planted, the body twists and the ligament pops. And/or the knee is hit by contact with another player, but this is usually not the case. Most ACL injuries happen without contact.

How many people suffer ACL injuries? What percentage are athletes?

There are up to 300,000 ACL injuries each year. About 70 percent occur during athletic participation.

How many young females suffer ACL injuries? What percentage of total female athletes?

Specific numbers are not available, but many sources say females suffer ACL injuries at a much greater rate than males.

Who is predisposed? Are some girls more prone to ACL injuries?

Girls in general have a greater chance of suffering an ACL injury than boys, and there are a number of explanations. Girls have wider hips. The thigh bone reaches the knee at a greater angle than it does in boys who enjoy a more straight up and down alignment. And female hip sockets are further forward. For those two reasons female feet roll inward and cause stress to the knee. Females also have looser knee joints, more flexible hamstrings, smaller ACLs, less muscle development and athletic prowess (boys generally start athletics earlier) and different hormones that affect things.

Maybe it's a difficult thing to say out loud, but it's probably true: The more boyish the build (slim hips aligned over knees and feet, strong core and legs) — the better suited young females will be to make athletic moves without knee injury.

How can the danger of injury be mitigated?

It has been suggested that girls need to learn how to move athletically at a younger age, something that perhaps comes more naturally to boys. Training begins with an athletic stance — bent at the waist and knees, balanced, on your toes ready to move in any direction. Girls must learn how to jump, land, stop and move with knees directly over the feet. They need to rehearse drills that emphasize proper stance and movement until it becomes more and more natural. At the same time they should develop strength to support the movement — especially in core (back and abs) and leg muscles.

How is an ACL repaired?

The ACL will not heal on its own. A strip of tissue must be surgically attached to replace the damaged ligament. The replacement tissue comes from the patellar, hamstring or quadriceps tendons. These are tendons running south of the kneecap, north of the kneecap and behind the kneecap, respectively. The tissue can come from the patient or a cadaver.

Who does the fixing?

An orthopedic surgeon. Orthopedics (or orthopaedics) is the line of surgery and treatment involving the musculoskeletal system — muscles, bones and connective tissue (tendons and ligaments).

What is surgery like?

It's pretty fast and efficient these days. (It used to be a game ender. Snap the ACL and one's playing days were over.) Now you do not spend the night in a hospital.

> At least with the surgery you are giving yourself another chance.

There is about an hour or so of preop, and then they guide you into surgery where you are promptly knocked out. The knee gets fixed, and you are wheeled into another room where you sleep it off.

When you wake, mom or dad will drive you home where you'll spend the rest of the day in a fog. You will receive a prescription for pain pills that you may need, but the pain shouldn't be too bad.

What the surgeon does

The procedure is called an ACL reconstruction. The damaged ligament is replaced with a graft using arthroscopic methods. The surgeon makes a small incision in your leg so that he can insert a small camera and light to see inside the knee. The image is projected onto a screen. Your surgeon will perform his work through small incisions around the knee.

Fun fact

The term arthroscopy derives from two Greek words, "arthro" (joint) and "skopein" (to look). It means "to look within the joint."

How long is recovery?

It seems like a very, very long time. Four to six weeks in a brace with crutches, six to nine months in a brace, and three months rehab. The latter is especially important for those who intend to return to athletics. Rehab is all about getting physically fit to play again.

What are the different stages of recovery like?

It takes focus and grit to remain positive and to recover successfully — there is no soft way through this thing. Crutches and brace are miserable. Throwing away the crutches is better, but stumbling around in a brace really sucks. Rehab is a lot of work if you are doing it right, but it gets better and better until one day you are ready to roll.

Will the repaired ACL be just as strong as my original ACL?

We found conflicting reports on what to expect. Many sources report that ACL surgery is usually a big success, and that the affected knee will be good to go. That's probably what your doctor is going to tell you. But we also ran across studies that suggest quite the opposite. Joy can say that while surgery got her back in the game, her second athletic career did not last long.

So it's iffy. Every individual case is different. But what else are you going to do? Without a new knee you will definitely be prone to further injury as well as osteoarthritis, and you won't be playing again. At least with the surgery you are giving yourself another chance.

After her second ACL injury, Joy will not be returning to a sport that requires cutting — planting a foot and changing direction with speed and power. But running is OK. As is sailing, paddling, hiking, swimming, maybe surfing and windsurfing ... a whole range of things. Her options are different now, but an active, outdoor life is still viable for sure.

Index

Acknowledgements

We are very grateful for the doctors who patched Joy up, Dr. Jonathan Myers and Dr. William Eves. The outfit that rehabbed Joy the first time, Rehab United, put Joy back in the game and how. Dr. Justin Balleza did the same the second time around and proved invaluable as a contributor to this book. Mark Hatmaker and Kylie Hatmaker graciously lent us images and helpful reviews. Kathleen Wheeler, Joy's mom and my wife, is there always to review, report and build us up. Phyllis Carter is the only editor we've ever had for Tracks Publishing and the first reason my books do not read like gibberish. Debbie Gerlack provided Joy with a mighty mentorship for four years of high school, and she will never know how much that has meant to me (Ms. Gerlack was the one who put the wayward coach in his place and helped Joy through her ordeals). Cristina Byvik's illustrations are always among the best things about any of my projects. I think her work is usually the best thing about any of the publications she contributes to.

Thank you for being on our side.

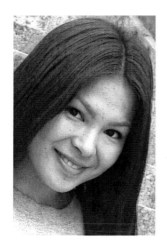

Joy Werner

Joy Werner graduated with honors from Hilltop High School in Chula Vista, California in 2015 and is now a student at UC Santa Barbara. She played club soccer in the San Diego area for several years and was a member of soccer, lacrosse and cross-country teams in high school.

Torn

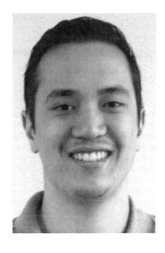

Dr. Justin Balleza, DPT

Dr. Justin Balleza was born and raised in the San Francisco Bay Area where he developed a passion for sports, fitness and biological sciences. Dr. Balleza pursued his interests and earned his B.S. in biology at the University of California, Riverside in 2010 and his Doctorate of Physical Therapy from the University of St. Augustine in 2013.

He has experience in treating a variety of orthopedic and neurological dysfunctions and utilizes an eclectic approach in patient care. He uses a wide variety of joint mobilizations, soft tissue release techniques and therapeutic exercise to get patients functioning at an optimal level. Dr. Balleza's life experience in competitive sports such as basketball, tennis and cycling as well as general fitness and athletic training allow him to apply specific and individualized therapy catered to each patient.

Torn

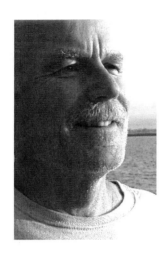

Doug Werner

Doug Werner is the founder of Tracks Publishing and Start-Up Sports®. He is the author of all eleven books in the Start-Up Sports series® and co-author of several other sport instructional guides including *Fitness Training for Girls* and *Beautiful Soccer*. He lives in Chula Vista, California with wife Kathleen and a dog named Blue.

Torn

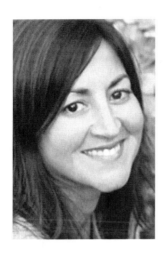

Cristina Byvik

Cristina Byvik is the chief illustrator for the *San Diego Union-Tribune.* She has won several awards from the Society of News Design, *Print Magazine* and the National Headliner Awards. Her work has appeared in a number of books and major publications including the *Washington Post.* She lives in Encinitas, California with husband, Kevin and son, Owen.

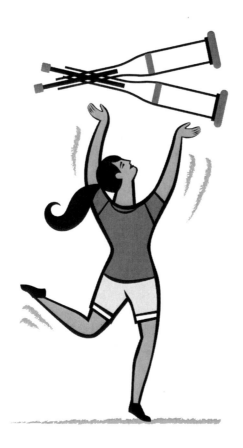